Using Cost-Effectiveness Analysis
to Improve Health Care

USING
COST-EFFECTIVENESS ANALYSIS
TO IMPROVE HEALTH CARE

Opportunities and Barriers

. . . .

Peter J. Neumann

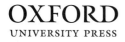

OXFORD
UNIVERSITY PRESS

2005

OXFORD
UNIVERSITY PRESS

Oxford   New York
Auckland   Bangkok   Buenos Aires   Cape Town   Chennai
Dar es Salaam   Delhi   Hong Kong   Istanbul   Karachi   Kolkata
Kuala Lumpur   Madrid   Melbourne   Mexico City   Mumbai   Nairobi
São Paulo   Shanghai   Taipei   Tokyo   Toronto

Copyright © 2005 by Oxford University Press, Inc.

Published by Oxford University Press, Inc.
198 Madison Avenue, New York, New York 10016

www.oup.com

Oxford is a registered trademark of Oxford University Press

Library of Congress Cataloging-in-Publication Data
Neumann, Peter J., 1961–
Using cost-effectiveness analysis to improve health care: opportunities and barriers /
Peter J. Neumann.
p. cm.
ISBN 0-19-517186-1
1. Medical care—Cost effectiveness.   2. Medical care, Cost of.   3. Cost effectiveness.
I. Title.
RA410.5.N48 2004
362.1'068'1—dc22   2004049244

9 8 7 6 5 4 3 2 1

Printed in the United States of America
on acid-free paper

To Hildy, Ariel, and Anna

Preface

. . . .

Does the world need another book on cost-effectiveness analysis (CEA) in health care?

It already has a number of excellent ones, including widely read how-to manuals (Drummond et al., 1997), a popular "bible" on the topic by the U.S. Panel on Cost-Effectiveness in Health and Medicine (Gold et al., 1996), and numerous volumes that address theoretical and methodological issues and advances (e.g., Johannesson, 1996; Nord, 1999; Pettiti, 2000; Drummond and McGuire, 2001).

Furthermore, does anyone in the United States really use cost-effectiveness analysis? The question has been posed frequently, even (or especially) by analysts themselves but then left hanging, shrugged off like a remark about the weather or the latest impasse in the Middle East.

Despite its promise and the steady stream of analyses conducted and published, policy makers in the United States have shied away from using CEA openly. This experience contrasts markedly with the flourishing application of CEA to coverage and reimbursement decisions abroad.

Why? The usual explanation—that Americans are different, that we are rugged individualists who will not accept explicit rationing—seems too convenient and too simplistic, and anyway not at all helpful. Why are CEAs being published widely in mainstream American medical journals if the technique is hopelessly ineffectual? Are there examples in which American policy makers have successfully applied the approach? What can we learn from them?

CEA offers a powerful tool to help prioritize resources for health care more efficiently. As health spending in the United States soars past $1.5 trillion, CEA lies at the heart of perhaps the ultimate health policy question: how can we get good value for our money?

I have been wondering about resistance to CEA in the United States for many years. A formative experience was a two-year stint in the early 1990s working at the Health Care Financing Administration (HCFA), the federal agency that administers the Medicare and Medicaid programs (the agency has since been renamed the "Centers for Medicare and Medicaid Services" [CMS]). Medicare at the time was trying to incorporate cost-effectiveness analysis formally into its procedures for covering new medical technology. The rationale seemed overwhelmingly sound, given escalating health spending, the diffusion of expensive new technologies, and the aging population. So did the timing: cost-effectiveness analysis was moving into mainstream journals and onto the minds of serious policy makers. And yet Medicare stumbled and to this day has never included CEA formally in its procedures.

I had addressed the topic cursorily in a paper or two over the years, but a comprehensive and (I hoped) fresh treatment seemed worth undertaking. With Medicare's experience as the catalyst, I set out to understand America's resistance to CEA, and to offer advice to CEA practitioners and policy makers for the future. This book is the product of those inquiries.

The chapters themselves are organized around an effort to understand this resistance and to build a case for the way forward. Chapter 2 provides a brief history of CEA in the United States. It discusses the roots of CEA in health and medicine, its promise for rational resource allocation, and its promotion to the medical community.

Chapter 3 explores the nature of the opposition to CEA, describing the antagonism CEA has encountered at public and private health programs across the nation.

Chapter 4 considers explanations for the resistance, including a lack of understanding about the conceptual approach, mistrust of the methodology, and mistrust of the motives of researchers and their sponsors.

Chapter 5 analyzes legal, regulatory, and political barriers to CEA, and includes a discussion of the ethical debate surrounding its applications.

Chapter 6 takes on the Oregon experience and the dos and don'ts it provides for American policy makers.

Chapter 7 documents how CEA has shaped health care decision-making in the United States, even in the face of resistance. It argues that CEA has actually enjoyed influence in the United States, not as an explicit instrument for prioritizing health services, but as a subtle lever on policy discourses. The chapter first reconciles hostility towards CEA with the rapid growth of analyses in mainstream American medical journals. It then reviews ways in which various policy makers in the public and private sectors have managed to incorporate CEA, sometimes under the radar screen, into their internal processes.

Chapter 8 turns to decision makers overseas who have incorporated CEA into their coverage and reimbursement deliberations. It reviews the experience of the United Kingdom's National Institute of Clinical Excellence, the recently created health authority with a broad mandate to issue guidance on the effectiveness and cost-effectiveness of health technologies and the clinical management of specific conditions. The chapter also discusses the experiences of public authorities in other nations, particularly Australia and Canada, which have formalized the use of CEA in resource allocation considerations.

In chapter 9 the book looks ahead. First, it anticipates the way forward by providing a perspective on what we have learned in 25 years of cost-effectiveness research. Second, it imagines a future for CEA that includes the prospects for change and a roadmap for getting there.

Chapter 10 offers pragmatic advice for practitioners. It discusses ways in which analysts can better translate their research by altering the manner in which they frame and present studies, by considering their audience more carefully, and by changing the language they use to describe their results. The chapter also discusses the importance of considering "affordability" alongside cost-effectiveness ratios.

Chapter 11 presents advice for the policy maker and politician. It provides a series of take-home lessons: CEA should not be used rigidly; it does not mean cost-containment; separate analysts from decision-makers; how you say it counts; process matters; raise the C/E threshold; incentives come first; and think broadly across sectors. It also considers the need for leadership at local, state, and national levels. If Americans are to enjoy better health in relation to the resources expended, leadership will be needed to provide the vision and to establish the conditions for change.

Acknowledgments

. . . .

I am grateful to many people for their support, advice, and encouragement. Milton Weinstein has provided wise counsel and unfailingly good mentorship for over 15 years. He encouraged me to undertake this project in the first place and also read an early draft and provided many good suggestions.

Jeffrey House, of Oxford University Press, provided first-rate editorial advice from the very outset. The book is greatly improved for his input and the gracious manner in which it was delivered.

The Dean's office at the Harvard School of Public Health granted a semester-long junior faculty sabbatical, which freed me from some day-to-day responsibilities and provided invaluable time to devote to this effort.

This book draws upon research I have conducted over the past seven years. I am grateful for support during that time from the National Science Foundation, the Agency for Health Care Research and Quality, and the Robert Wood Johnson Foundation.

I am also thankful for specific permission to draw upon my previously published material. Sections of Chapter 4 are drawn from "Paying the Piper for Pharmacoeconomic Studies," in Medical Decision Making, 1998. Material in Chapter 6 stems from two previous papers in *Health Affairs*, "The FDA's regulation of health economic information" (2000, with Karl Claxton and Milton Weinstein) and "Evidence-based and value-based formulary guidelines" (2004). Parts of Chapters 1 and 9 are drawn from my paper (with Sue Goldie and Milton Weinstein) "Preference-based measures for economic evaluation," in the *Annual Review of Public Health* (2000). Chapters 8 and 10 contain excerpts from "Why Don't Americans Use Cost-Effectiveness Analysis?" at the *American Journal of Managed Care* (2004).

An outstanding team of researchers have worked to assemble and analyze the registry of cost-effectiveness analyses (www.hsph.harvard.edu/cearegistry) upon which some of this book is drawn. I have been privileged to work with Chaim Bell, Richard Chapman, Dan Greenberg, Peijung Lin, Natalia Olchanski, Mandy Patrick, Allison Rosen, Eileen Sandberg, and Pat Stone.

Dan Greenberg and Nomita Divi read drafts of the entire manuscript and gave me a great deal of valuable feedback on matters large and small. I have also benefited from conversations with others at the Harvard School of Public Health, including Norman Daniels, David Hemenway, Michelle Mello, and David Studdert.

I have profited greatly from being around many wonderful colleagues at the Harvard Center for Risk Analysis over the years, including John Graham, the former director, who brought me there in the first place, and numerous others: Josh Cohen, Sue Goldie, George Gray, Jim Hammitt, Karen Kuntz, David Ropeik, and scores of talented and energetic students.

My parents, brothers, and entire extended family have always been terrifically supportive, and I thank them heartily.

Finally, I am forever indebted to my wife, Hildy, and daughters, Ariel and Anna, to whom this book is dedicated, for their endless love and patience.

Contents

. . . .

Using Cost-Effectiveness Analysis
to Improve Health Care

1

Introduction

. . . .

> *Ruin is the destination toward which all men rush, each pursuing his own*
> *best interest in a society that believes in the freedom of the commons.*
> *Freedom in a commons brings ruin to all.*
>
> —Garrett Hardin, 1968

Cost-effectiveness analysis (CEA) logically should occupy an important place
in the health policy-making toolkit. It offers decision makers a structured,
rational approach to improve the return on resources expended. But decades after its widespread promotion to the medical community, policy
makers in the United States remain reluctant to use the approach formally.
Indeed, the resistance to economic evidence in the United States in an era
of evidence-based medicine in health care is perhaps the most notable
development of all.

The lack of scrutiny of this phenomenon is also noteworthy. Despite the
pervasiveness of economic evaluations in the public health and medical
literature, researchers have devoted little attention to understanding how
and when decision makers use the technique, why they do *not* use it, and
how experience can guide better policies for the future.

This book attempts to fill that void. It is motivated by the thought that
an inquiry into the uses and non-uses of CEA will yield important lessons
about the nature of the resistance, and about ways to advance the field.

A secondary impetus is the idea that how a nation uses CEA offers a
prism through which to understand the collective values underlying its
health-care system. The general resistance to CEA in the United States,
and the way it has been fashioned to satisfy political realities in the few
instances where it has been applied (e.g., in the Oregon Medicaid program),
provide broader lessons for health policy makers. So, too, do the experiences of Europe, Canada, and Australia, where CEA enjoys more widespread acceptance.

Leading works on CEA typically underscore the idea that health policy makers should not use it in a mechanical way, and that cost-effectiveness is but one of many inputs into health policy decisions (Gold et al., 1996 p. 10). *The U.S. Panel on Cost-Effectiveness in Health and Medicine* (the *Panel*) emphasizes, for example, that "cost-effectiveness analyses are an aid to decision making, not a complete procedure for making decisions, because they cannot incorporate all the values relevant to the decisions" (Gold et al., 1996, p. 22).

The matter is generally left there, however, without serious exploration of these values, or of the practical hurdles facing decision makers. Some observers have discussed aspects of the resistance, emphasizing that CEA ignores the working needs of actual health-care managers (Langley, 2000; Prosser et al., 2000), or stressing the ethical (Nord, 1999; Ubel, 2000; Daniels and Sabin, 2002), political (Brown, 1991; Jacobs et al., 1999), or legal (Jacobson and Kanna, 2001) dilemmas that the technique poses.

This book attempts a fuller treatment by placing the resistance front and center in order to analyze explicitly the influences of other factors along-side cost-effectiveness information, as a means towards advancing the field. In doing so, I seek to provide a unique perspective among cost-effective-ness studies.

Existing works on CEA generally concentrate on methods and concepts, targeting those who conduct or appraise analyses (e.g., Gold et al.,1996; Haddix et al., 1996; Drummond et al., 1997a). In contrast, the adjacent space on the bookshelf for related matters of politics and policy is sparsely settled. The few works that consider the practice of using cost-effectiveness cover the European experience (e.g., Pinto et al., 2001). Moreover, these books are edited volumes, which tend to give snapshots rather than a pano-rama. This book attempts to provide a narrative that captures the whole U.S. experience.

Emphatically, my intent is not to address theoretical debates about the measurement of "future" costs or discount rates, or about which compo-nents belong in the numerator or denominator of the cost-effectiveness ratio. Those debates rage on elsewhere (e.g., Brouwer et al., 1998; Meltzer and Johannesson, 1999; Garber, 1999; Russell, 1999; Weinstein, 1999). Rather, my aim is to review the historical record and uncover the lessons it reveals about cost-effectiveness analysis, and to offer advice for practitioners and policy makers.

The question whether anyone really uses cost-effectiveness analysis in the United States has been posed in papers and at conferences over the years (e.g., Power and Eisenberg, 1998). To ask this question itself betrays a certain amount of insecurity in the field, and a measure of yearning. (Do we have conferences on whether health policy makers use epidemiology, statistics, or economics?) The question does, however, reflect the genuine unfriendliness the technique has encountered.

The Panel on Cost-Effectiveness in Health and Medicine states that CEA should be of use to managed care organizations, insurers, health departments, and state and federal policy makers (Gold et al., 1996, p. xxii), as well as secondary audiences such as clinical guideline developers, benefits managers, patient advocacy groups, the press, and the general public (Gold et al., 1996, pp. 55–58). It stresses the need for cost-effectiveness analysts to take into account the real policy contexts and controversies that relate to decisions about the use of a program, and to have an idea about how a study will actually contribute to decisions (Gold et al., 1996, p. 55).

In fact, the *Panel* and other leading works (e.g., Haddix et al., 1996) devote little attention to actual contexts and controversies. They seldom consider the public and private institutions involved, or the organizational or political constraints confronting decision makers.

The U.S. Medicare program's experience with CEA offers a prime example. As perhaps the world's largest single payer of health services, and one perennially facing budgetary shortfalls, the program should be an enthusiastic consumer of cost-effectiveness information. Instead, after repeated attempts to incorporate cost-effectiveness formally as a criterion for covering new medical technologies, Medicare has eschewed formal use of this technique, a development that has received remarkably little attention in the CEA field. In recent years, Medicare has avoided cost-effectiveness even as it has restructured its entire apparatus for covering new technologies in an attempt to make its process more transparent, consistent, and evidence-based (*U.S. Federal Register*, 1998 and 1999). Medicare's retreat from cost-effectiveness also defies the federal government's broader movement to subject new regulations to formal cost-benefit and cost-effectiveness tests (Hahn, 2002; Office of Management and Budget (OMB), 2003).

The Oregon Medicaid program's effort to prioritize health services offers another example. Oregon initially sought to rank services based on their cost-effectiveness. But the plan was opposed on legal, political, and ethical grounds, and was implemented only after the offending cost-effectiveness provisions were removed. Unlike Medicare's experience with cost-effectiveness, Oregon's received a great deal of attention from scholars. However, the focus from cost-effectiveness experts has generally been parochial—that Oregon's prioritization scheme never reflected actual cost-effectiveness in the first place (Tengs et al., 1996), or that explanations can be found in the plan's lack of methodological rigor (Gold et al., 1996, p. vii), or that its use of quality-adjusted life-years gained (QALYs) failed to capture true public preferences about rationing health care (Ubel et al., 1996). The enduring lessons of Oregon are larger, political ones. No other state Medicaid program in the nation tried to emulate Oregon's plan or fix its technical problems.

Why have managed-care plans not embraced CEA? Given their turbulent finances and their professed desire to enhance value by coordinating health care, one might expect them to be eager consumers of cost-effectiveness information. Instead, studies suggest that they resist explicit use of the information. When asked in surveys, for example, health plan officials say that cost-effectiveness does not play a role in decision-making, or that it is a minor, secondary consideration after clinical factors (e.g., Luce et al., 1996; Titlow et al., 2000). Health plans *have* embraced many management tools in an attempt to deliver care more efficiently, from restrictive formularies to risk-sharing arrangements with physicians. Why then do they recoil from CEA?

While offering a marvelous recipe for resource allocation, CEA seems to have fallen short as a pragmatic program. Clinical guidelines tend to ignore cost-effectiveness information (Wallace et al., 2002). Indeed, studies find little relationship at all between the cost-effectiveness of interventions and their actual implementation (Tengs and Graham, 1996).

Is there something inherently problematic about the approach? Curiously, the *Panel* recognizes the failure even as it champions the technique, noting "there is little indication . . . that cost-effectiveness analysis contributes systematically to resource allocation decisions in United States medicine," but that, on the contrary, evidence suggests that decision makers don't use costs, and are reluctant to limit care explicitly (Gold et al., 1996, p. 19).

In exploring the disconnection between the promise of CEA and the persistent failure of rational intentions, this book's objective is to find common ground and practical solutions. My premise is that policy makers should use formal techniques to evaluate tradeoffs and help society invest its health resources wisely.

Proponents of CEA have sometimes defended the methodology by noting that the technique is still a new kid on the block (e.g., Eddy, 1992; Ubel, 2000). The problem with this argument is that after 25 years, CEA's formative years are behind it.

Recognizing the public's resistance to explicit consideration of limits, some have called for honest debate about rationing (e.g., Ubel, 2000; Daniels et al., 2002). This book calls also for a political one. That is, the way forward is not simply a matter of owning up to society's need to ration. Rather, it lies in understanding the political nature of the resistance and in fashioning strategies that overcome or perhaps accommodate it.

In this sense, my book is both descriptive and prescriptive. It offers practical advice to analysts and decision makers. For practitioners, the book provides recommendations about how to improve the translation of CEAs. For policy makers, it presents a series of guideposts to direct the implementation of CEA. It also tries to anticipate specific future policy struggles. The audience, I hope, will include students taking health policy courses in schools of public health, medicine, or business; cost-effectiveness analysts working in business, government, or academia; and health outcomes managers within the pharmaceutical industry or managed-care industries.

There are a few encouraging signs for CEA. Examples in the United States include the promulgation and adoption of new guidelines from drug formulary committees, which request drug manufacturers to submit economic evidence to formulary committees (Neumann, 2004). Another is the recent decision by the U.S. Task Force on Preventive Services to consider cost-effectiveness in its recommendations. In Europe, Canada, and Australia, open consideration of the cost-effectiveness of new pharmaceuticals has become a routine feature of reimbursement deliberations. The World Health Organization has launched an ambitious project to provide decision makers with cost-effectiveness evidence for purposes of setting priorities and improving the performance of health systems (World Health Organization, 2003). However, where use of cost-effectiveness information has emerged, it has done so, not as the Oregon plan's architects envisioned, but in a more nuanced fashion.

A note about terminology at the outset. Economic evaluations of healthcare interventions can take a number of forms. Many are *cost-analyses* or *cost-identification analyses*, which simply estimate and compare the net costs of different strategies. For example, analysts might compare the net costs (costs of the drug and associated side effects minus any cost offsets) of chemotherapy for lung cancer versus best supportive care. A limitation of this approach, however, is that it does not explicitly consider health outcomes. Analysts sometimes tailor cost analyses for particular audiences. For example, cost analyses may be conducted by managed-care plans to determine the impact of a new drug on its internal budget, or the impact of a new drug on enrollees "per member per month" (Campen, 2002). Other analysts may present the impact of new drug on societal costs, which include direct costs (the value of the goods, services, and other resources consumed in the provision of an intervention), as well as patient time costs (the value of the time a patient spends seeking care or participating in a treatment) and productivity costs (the costs associated with lost or impaired ability to work) (Gold et al., 1996, pp. 179–181).

Another form, termed *cost-consequences analysis*, involves computing and listing components of costs and consequences of alternative programs, without any attempt to aggregate results into a single measure. Researchers conducting an economic evaluation of a new antidepressant, for instance, might evaluate the net costs (total costs minus any savings produced) and health effects (in terms of the percent change on a validated depression scale) compared to an alternative treatment strategy. A limitation of the approach is that it does not permit comparisons across diverse diseases or conditions. For example, how can one compare the value of a drug for depression with the value of a drug for angina?

An alternative approach is cost-benefit analysis (CBA), in which all costs and benefits are measured and compared in monetary terms. The requirement for monetary valuation of health benefits in CBA (e.g., valuing life-years saved at $100,000 each), however, raises measurement challenges and political objections.

In recent years, cost-effectiveness analysis has emerged as the recommended analytical technique for conducting economic evaluation of health and medical interventions (Gold et al., 1996). The appeal of this approach is that it allows a convenient means of quantifying both economic and health benefits in a single ratio. Cost-effectiveness analyses involve comparisons between two alternatives, or between the presence and absence of an intervention: the cost per effect (C/E) ratio reflects the increment or difference in the interventions' costs divided by the difference in their health effectiveness (Gold et al., 1996).

While cost-effectiveness analyses can measure health effects in disease-specific terms (e.g., costs per number of cancer cases prevented), a growing trend is to evaluate interventions using a standard measurement, which permits comparisons across diverse interventions and diseases. One way to standardize ratios is to measure health effects in terms of life expectancy—the cost-effectiveness ratio for each alternative would reflect the costs per *year of life gained*. A limitation of this approach is that life expectancy alone does not take into account the quality of additional time that is gained (for instance, an added month of life with disability or pain is valued the same as an added month without disability or pain). Ideally, an analysis would capture such effects.

The approach recommended by the Panel on Cost-Effectiveness, as well as other consensus groups, is to measure health outcomes in terms of "quality-adjusted" life years (QALYs) (Gold et al., 1996; Menon et al., 1996). QALYs represent the benefit of a health intervention as time spent in a series of "quality-weighted" health states, where the quality weights reflect the desirability of living in the state, typically from "perfect" health (weighted 1.0) to death (weighted 0.0). Researchers have used a number of techniques over the years to construct these quality weights. One option is to use "standard gamble" or "time tradeoff" techniques, which have a sound theoretical basis in economic utility theory. These methods involve asking respondents to value health states by explicitly considering how much they would be willing to sacrifice to avoid being in a particular health state. Alternative elicitation techniques include rating scales in which respondents are asked to express the strength of their preferences for particular health states by marking a point on a scale.

Once the quality weights are obtained for each state, they are multiplied by the time spent in the state; these products are summed to obtain the total number of quality-adjusted life years. The advantage of using QALYs is twofold: they capture in a single measure gains from both prolongation and improved quality of life, and they incorporate the value or preferences people place on different outcomes (Drummond et al., 1997).

The Panel on Cost-Effectiveness in Health and Medicine was charged with "assessing the current state of the science of the field, and with providing recommendations for the conduct of studies in order to improve their quality and encourage their comparability" (Gold et al., 1996). Among other recommendations, the Panel proposed the use of a *reference case*, a standard set of methodological practices that an analyst would seek to follow in a cost-effectiveness analysis (CEA) if results from different studies are to be compared (Russell et al., 1996; Weinstein et al., 1996). For example, the Panel recommends that cost-effectiveness analysts should clearly identify the intervention under investigation as well as the comparator being studied and the target population. It also urges analysts to be transparent about the study perspective, the time horizon, and the precise methods used for measuring costs and health benefits. Importantly, the Panel recommended that the reference case use QALYs to identify and assign value to health outcomes.

A common practice among analysts conducting cost-per-life-year or cost-per-QALY ratios is to rank the ratios in *league tables*, in which interventions are ranked by their incremental cost-effectiveness. League tables provide a convenient means of furnishing information about how to allocate health resources efficiently among many competing health interventions— lower C/E ratios reflect more efficient ways to produce QALYs.

For convenience, I use the term *cost-effectiveness analysis* in this book generally to mean a formal economic evaluation of a health-care technology, service, or program. Many political and policy discussions about the use of economic evaluations refer generically to "cost-effectiveness analysis" without restricting the focus to cost per life-year or cost per QALY analyses per se. Where the distinctions among the actual technique are important and more precise terms warranted, I call attention to them. Readers interested in learning more about conceptual and methodological issues surrounding cost-effectiveness analysis should consult one or more of several excellent references on the topic (e.g., Gold et al., 1996; Johannesson, 1996; Drummond et al., 1997).

2

The Promise and Promotion of CEA

. . . .

> *We believe that a disciplined effort to assess systematically the cost-effectiveness of technologies under coverage review will be useful. . . . Regular application of these principles . . . would vastly improve our knowledge base and be a deterrent to coverage of procedures that may be costly, but have little or no impact on improving health outcomes.*
> —U.S. Health Care Financing Administration, 1989

The Evolution of CEA

Some scholars attribute the intellectual roots of economic evaluation to the work of the French economist Jules Dupuit in the 1840s, though they note that theoretical development of the approach came decades later (Dupuit, 1844, cited in Arrow, 1988). However, the first formal application of cost-benefit/cost-effectiveness analysis may have been by Richard Petty, who argued two centuries earlier for greater social investment in medicine on grounds that the value of a saved human life exceeds the cost of investment (Warner and Luce, 1982). Researchers also point to recommendations of U.S. Secretary of the Treasury Albert Gallatin in 1808 to compare the costs and benefits of water-related projects (Hanley and Spash, 1993), and to Lemuel Shattuck, who used similar arguments to appeal for sanitary reforms in Boston in the mid–nineteenth century (Warner and Luce, 1982).

The first legislation to apply formal cost-benefit/cost-effectiveness analysis in the United States came in 1902 with the River and Harbor Act, which required the U.S. Army Corps of Engineers to assess the costs and benefits of river and harbor projects (Office of Technology Assessment [OTA], (1994). This was followed by the Flood Control Act of 1936, which required the U.S. Bureau of Reclamation to assess its water projects and stipulated that "benefits [of projects] to whomsoever they may accrue [must be] in excess of the estimated costs," though no guidance was provided on how to measure benefits and costs (Hanley and Spash, 1993; OTA, 1994).

Applications of CEA/CBA from the 1930s to the 1960s included those by the Tennessee Valley Authority, the Department of Agriculture, and especially by the Defense Department under Secretary Robert McNamara in the 1960s, which adopted a budgeting system that used CEA to evaluate alternative defense programs (Warner and Luce, 1982). The logic of CEA was incorporated into an initiative by President Johnson in the 1960s to rationalize government resource allocation (Schultze, 1968; Rivlin, 1971) and left a legacy of systematic thinking and rational analysis in government decision-making (Warner and Luce, 1982). Important scholarly developments in the era that helped provide the intellectual foundation for CEA include work by Eckstein (1958) on benefit estimation, by Arrow (1963) on the welfare economics of medical care, and by Raiffa (1968) on the prescriptive methodology of decision analysis (cited in Hanley and Spash, 1993; and Gold et al., 1996).

In the 1960s and early 1970s, health officials at the U.S. Department of Health, Education, and Welfare began applying CEA to a variety of health problems, including kidney disease and maternal and child health programs (e.g., Klarman, 1968). Warner and Luce (1982) note that the Health Planning Amendments of 1979 and Health Care Technology Act of 1978 called for inclusion of cost-effectiveness in the deliberative processes of the agencies affected.

In the 1970s and early 1980s, cost-effectiveness analyses of health problems began to appear in major medical journals, including influential papers examining the cost-effectiveness of inexpensive tests for cancer screening (Neuhauser and Lewicki, 1975; Eddy 1980b), of strategies to manage hypertension (Stason and Weinstein, 1976), and of vaccines for pneumococcal pneumonia (Sisk et al., 1980). Articles in the *New England Journal of Medicine* discussed the tension between finite resources for health care amidst ever-growing demands (Hiatt, 1975), the appeal of formal CEA to address the problem (Weinstein and Stason, 1977), and the link between cost-effectiveness analysis and health technology assessment (Fineberg and Hiatt, 1979). In 1982 authors of a book on the topic stated confidently that CEA "represents an idea whose time has come" (Warner and Luce, 1982).

The Promise of CEA

The emergence of CEA in health care in the 1960s and 1970s represented a paradigm shift. For one thing it reflected the growing awareness that American medicine had exceeded society's capacity to pay for all of the health care that people could use to actually improve their health (Weinstein and Stason, 1977).

This was a watershed period for American medicine, one characterized by new concerns about escalating health costs. Paul Starr, in *The Social Transformation of American Medicine*, notes that the key concern that had guided medicine until that time was that Americans needed *more* medical care—more than the marketplace would provide by itself (Starr, pp. 379–80). By the 1970s, however, concerns about costs were replacing concerns about expanding access. The nation's focus turned to the problem of unnecessary procedures, excessive rates of surgery and hospitalization, and duplication of facilities and equipment (Starr, 1982, p. 383). The cost of medical services rose from an average annual rate of 3.2% in the seven years preceding the enactment of Medicare and Medicaid in 1965 to 7.9% in years afterward (overall inflation jumped from 2.0 to 5.8 during the same time period). From 1970 to 1980, health-care expenditures jumped from $69 million to $230 billion, an increase from 7.2% to 9.4% of the gross national product (GNP) (U.S. Public Health Service, 1981, cited in Starr, 1982, pp. 380, 384).

The appearance of CEA and related techniques signaled the growing appeal of scientific and "rational" approaches to social problems, including health problems. Starr (1982, p. 381) observes that the crisis over costs in health care also bred optimism about the possibilities for reform. To CEA's proponents, the possibilities were clear. Efficiency was an article of faith. Without such aids, we would make serious errors in judgment. Misallocations, distortions, and haphazard spending in the portfolio of investments to improve health were inevitable (Weinstein and Stason, 1977; Graham and Vaupel, 1981; Morral, 1986).

We already ration health care in hidden ways—the logic went—better to do it rationally. CEA would help policy makers apportion society's scarce health resources. Rather than allowing 15% of Americans to go without health insurance, we could cover all citizens and achieve more overall health improvement by foregoing uses of health care with little or no marginal benefit and by redirecting resources towards more effective opportunities.

CEA represented a way to level the playing field and to bring structure and order and scientific reasoning to an unruly and inequitable health care system. Its decision-analytical underpinnings gave policy makers a framework for posing a range of questions related to priority-setting (Gold et al., 1996, p. xviii). It allowed them to compare existing alternatives, explore hypothetical strategies, and test the strength of underlying assumptions, all in an explicit, quantitative, and systematic way (Haddix et al., p. 27; Gold et al., 1998, pp. xix, 10–11). The process represented a profound change for a health community conditioned to thinking about medical needs, and unaccustomed to contemplating tradeoffs explicitly.

Over the years, CEA in health care was shaped by multiple disciplines, including medicine, public health, sociology, psychology, epidemiology, ethics, and economics (Gold et al., 1996, pp. xvii, 25). Economists provided a theoretical framework, emphasizing economic principles and social welfare (Garber and Phelps, 1995). As the Panel noted, formal CEA became not simply a mathematical technique to explain how one could optimize resources, but a normative theory about how one *should* do so (Gold et al., 1996, pp. 26, 37–38).

At its heart, however, CEA has remained a pragmatic approach, closer to its applied engineering and decision-analytical roots (Gold, pp. 25, 50). Leaders in the field have placed greater emphasis on providing decision makers with a practical tool than on remaining faithful to economic doctrine per se.

The influence of the pragmatists is evident in the field's recent preference for CEA over cost-benefit analysis (CBA), despite the latter's early popularity and its stronger foundations in economic theory.

Health policy analysts traditionally used CBA to assess the value of health programs (Weisbrod, 1961). In CBA, analysts estimate the net social benefit of a program or intervention as the incremental benefit of a program minus the incremental cost. All costs and benefits are measured in monetary units (e.g., dollars). The approach is useful because it leads to a simple decision rule: if a program's net benefits exceed its net costs, then it should be adopted. CBA, however, also raises measurement difficulties in that it requires the monetary valuation of health benefits. That is, how should we value, in dollar terms, a case of cancer avoided or a life saved?

Early on, cost-benefit analysts quantified health benefits with a "human capital" approach. The value of reduced health was measured as the lost earnings of affected individuals. The advantage of the human capital approach was that it approximated value as the "productive potential" of society lost through morbidity and mortality. It also permitted a relatively straightforward calculation. The disadvantage, as critics such as Schelling (1968) and Mishan (1971) noted, is that the approach has no basis in economic theory—because it ignores underlying consumer preferences and implies that unproductive periods such as leisure time and retirement were without value.

A superior approach would acknowledge that consumers make tradeoffs between health and other goods and services. People don't spend all of their money to relieve their symptoms or to reduce their risk of death; instead, they consume to the point at which the improvement justifies the costs. Therefore, health should be valued by determining how much individuals are willing to pay for it. Unlike human capital, willingness-to-pay measures are preference-based. The metric is monetary, which allows tradeoffs with costs and non–health consequences.

A number of researchers have attempted to measure the value of health by assessing what people are willing to pay for specific health benefits. Economists typically measure the value of commodities by examining the prices of goods and services bought and sold in the marketplace. But since private markets for health benefits do not generally exist, it is difficult and often impossible to measure the value of health by appealing to market data. Therefore researchers have turned to other measures. Some have taken "revealed preference" approaches by imputing willingness to pay from comparable market prices or wages (e.g., the willingness to accept occupational risk could be valued as the incremental wage paid to such workers [Viscusi, 1993]). The problem is that prices and wages may not be truly comparable (i.e., unique properties of risk and benefit associated with a job may be confounded with the magnitude of the risk itself [Pauly, 1995]).

Others have used direct surveys of consumers, called *willingness-to-pay* or *contingent valuation* surveys because responses are contingent upon a hypothetical market for the good or service of interest (e.g., Acton, 1974; Johannesson and Jonsson, 1991; Neumann and Johannesson, 1994; O'Brien et al., 1996). The advantage of the approach is that it is grounded explicitly on principles of welfare economics, and provides a means to quantify the benefits of difficult-to-estimate factors such as the psychological benefits of symptom relief. The disadvantage is that researchers have often found that the method does not produce reliable estimates (Stahlhammer and Johannesson, 1996).

In recent years, cost-effectiveness analysis has emerged as a favored analytical technique for economic evaluation in health care. The major appeal of cost-effectiveness over cost-benefit analysis is that it allows analysts to quantify health benefits in "health" rather than in monetary terms. Consensus groups have emphasized the practical and political advantages of using CEA because valuing outcomes in dollars as CBA requires presents measurement difficulties and ethical dilemmas. The Panel, for example, stated that "our interest in cost-effectiveness analysis derives largely from its broad acceptance within the health care field, in contrast to the skepticism that often greets cost-benefit analyses in that arena" (Gold et al., 1996, p. 28).

The number of published CEAs in health care has vastly outpaced the number of CBAs over the years (Fig. 2–1). Orthodox economists have been left to remark that valuing outcomes in terms of QALYs presents its own moral and technical challenges (Pauly, 1995), and to point out the "near" equivalence of CEA to CBA (Phelps and Mushlin, 1991).

Spreading the Gospel

But who would actually *use* cost-effectiveness analysis? The most obvious consumers were policy makers in charge of allocating health resources. Proponents of CEA recognized early on, though, that success would also hinge on the technique's acceptance in the broader medical community. Practicing physicians needed to be converted, or at least neutralized as an opposing force.

This would require a shift in their thinking. Doctors had to begin contemplating limits, whereas their previous training emphasized the need to provide beneficial treatment or service without regard to the marginal costs.

Some of the challenges involved persuading physicians to acknowledge that they already rationed routinely, not explicitly but by "compromising" in varied and disguised ways—by not sending all post-operative patients to the intensive-care unit (ICU), by following health plan policies to give the most expensive drug only after others had failed, and by adhering to "standards of care," which recommended screening for cancer every, say, three years, rather than every two or one (Eddy, 1992a; Asch and Ubel, 1997; Ubel, 2000).

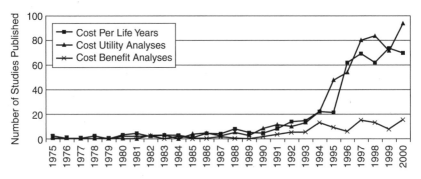

Figure 2–1. Trends in cost-effectiveness and cost–benefit analyses, 1975–2000. *Source*: OHE Health Economic Evaluations Database, 2003.

Beyond persuading physicians to concede the point, proponents wanted them to embrace CEA as the preferred rationing tool (Weinstein and Stason, 1977). A physician and mathematician, David Eddy, published a multi-series "Conversations with my Father," in the early 1990s in the *Journal of the American Medical Association*, which epitomized the trend to win over practicing physicians (Eddy 1992a–d). In his imagined conversation, Eddy patiently explains the technique to his elderly father, Maxon Eddy, M.D., who symbolizes the old-style American doctor—well-meaning, curmudgeonly, good-hearted, and stubborn. The elder Dr. Eddy stumbles along with the new concepts ("I think I follow you, but I'm not sure . . .") and eventually concedes that, yes, rationing is inevitable and that CEA offers opportunities, even as he hems and haws about its limitations. In the late 1980s and early 1990s—spurred largely by the debate over the Oregon health plan—leading medical journals began publishing pieces about rationing, with many (though not all) conceding a place for CEA as a useful tool for prioritization (e.g., Leaf, 1989).

In part, the arguments were practical. There were myriad things a physician could do in the course of a short office visit, and CEA provided a way to arrange competing priorities and deliver the greatest health benefit given the constraints.

Proponents, however, were also asking practicing physicians to explicitly consider their broader social obligations. Physicians had a collective duty to withhold health services that brought small additional benefits for their costs. CEA provided a way to ration fairly, deliberately, and openly. The other intended audience was the ever-expanding managerial ranks in health care, which included a growing number of hospital and health plan administrators, medical and pharmacy directors, and policy makers at public and private health institutions.

As national health spending continued to soar—from $246 billion (8.8% of gross domestic product [GDP] in 1980 to $1.4 trillion (14.1% of GDP) in 2000 (Centers for Medicare and Medicaid Services, 2004)—medical journals became conduits for broadcasting cost-effectiveness information. Elixhauser et al. (1993 and 1998) reported almost 3,000 economic evaluations of health-care interventions published from 1979 to 1996. The number of published cost-utility analyses (CUAs) rose from 10 in the 1980s to 270 in the 1990s, covering a wide range of conditions, intervention types, and treatment modalities (Neumann et al., 2000a; Greenberg and Pliskin, 2002; Neumann et al., in press). Between 1977 and 2001, the *Annals of Internal Medicine* published 29 CUAs, *Journal of the American Medical Association* 26, and *New England Journal of Medicine* 10 (Neumann et al., 2003).[1]

Other leading general medical and specialty journals were close behind.[2] Moreover, recommendations for conducting, reporting, and using such analyses were widely promoted to the medical community (Russell et al., 1996; Weinstein et al., 1996; Siegel et al., 1996; Drummond et al., 1997c; O'Brien et al., 1997). By the beginning of the twenty-first century, CEA had become a ubiquitous part of the medical culture.

3

Resistance to CEA in the United States

. . . .

> *It is apparent that cost-effectiveness analysis is extremely controversial for beneficiaries, providers, and suppliers. It raises fears of rationing based on cost. HCFA has not and does not intend to make coverage decisions based solely on cost-effectiveness, and we will not refuse to cover services merely because they are costly. Moreover, manufacturers or providers do not need to submit formal cost-effectiveness analyses to HCFA in order to have a service considered for coverage.*
> —Bruce Vladeck, Administrator of the U.S. Health Care Financing Administration, in testimony before Congress, 1997

> *If the technology was effective, we would find a way to pay for it. There is no dollar value per life per year at which Medicare would decline to pay.*
> —Sean Tunis, Director of Medicare's Coverage and Analysis Group, 2003

CEA's proponents have generally argued that a large part of CEA's appeal lies in its broad acceptability. Leading advocates have argued that CEA should be used to determine the content of medical care in most settings (e.g., Eddy 1992a). *The Panel on Cost-Effectiveness in Health and Medicine* notes that CEA could serve a range of masters, from a managed-care organization administrator who might wish to know the cost per year of life saved by a program for its enrolled population, to a state health official who might want to compare the cost per QALY gained of a blood lead-level treatment program to the cost per QALY gained of a program that improves the nutrition of school-age children (Gold et al., 1996, p. xviii). But a review of policies of public and private health-care payers in the United States reveals little support for the technique, and indeed active resistance in many cases.

The Medicare Experience

Medicare's statutory authority

Medicare's authorizing legislation in 1965 prohibits payment under Medicare for any expenses incurred for "items and services that are not reasonable and necessary for the diagnosis or treatment of illness or injury or to improve the functioning of a malformed body member" (1862(a)(1)(A) of Social Security Act).

The statute leaves a number of questions unanswered. While it restricts the universe of services covered—excluding cosmetic surgery, personal comfort items, custodial care, routine physical checkups, and outpatient drugs (*U.S. Federal Register*, 1989, p. 4304)—for practical reasons the statute does not provide an all-inclusive list of specific covered treatments. As Garber (2001) notes, it is not always clear what constitutes an illness or injury—the statute implies that Medicare would pay to treat memory loss but not to improve memory, for example.

Even more challenging is how to interpret which covered services are "reasonable and necessary." Some version of the "reasonable and necessary" clause was required given Medicare's role as a payer. Medicare could not simply enact a policy to cover all devices and inpatient drugs approved by the Food and Drug Administration (FDA). The FDA judges whether a new drug or device is safe and effective. A drug could be safe and effective and FDA-approved, but not reasonable and necessary, however—if, for example, it cost substantially more but offered no more benefits than an existing Medicare-covered drug (Garber, 2001). U.S. law stipulates that the FDA worry about the health risks and benefits of scientific advances, but that Medicare worry about paying for the advances.[1]

How does "reasonable and necessary" align with "cost-effective?" As Medicare's spending rose inexorably with the march of new technologies and favorable incentives in the program to use them, it was inevitable that Medicare would confront this question.

HCFA's 1989 proposed regulations. The Health Care Financing Administration (HCFA) (now called the Centers for Medicare and Medicaid Services [CMS]), which administers the Medicare program,[2] traditionally interpreted "reasonable and necessary" to mean "safe, effective, non-investigational and appropriate." Specifically, they based their decisions on whether a service was proven in scientific studies or generally accepted in the medical community as safe and effective for its intended use (*U.S. Federal Register*, 1989, pp. 4304–8). Because of the complexity and diversity of issues involved in making coverage decisions, Medicare did not, in the first two decades of the program, "think it is possible, or advisable, to try to set quantitative standards or develop a formula for the application of those criteria" (*U.S. Federal Register*, 1989, pp. 4304–8).

Emboldened by what the agency called an "explosion of high-cost medical technologies" (as well as other factors, including the broader movement towards evidence-based medicine, public pressure on Medicare to make its coverage criteria more understandable and transparent, and settlement of a court case[3]), HCFA proposed in 1989 to include cost-effectiveness as a criterion in deciding whether to cover new medical technologies (*U.S. Federal Register*, 1989, pp. 4304–8).

Asserting that costs were relevant in deciding whether to expand or continue coverage of technologies, HCFA explained that "We believe the requirement of section 1882(a)(1) that a covered service be "reasonable" encompasses the authority to consider cost as a factor in making Medicare coverage determinations" (*U.S. Federal Register*, 1989, p. 4308).

HCFA argued that a disciplined effort to assess systematically the cost-effectiveness of technologies under coverage review would "vastly improve our knowledge base and be a deterrent to coverage of procedures that may be costly, but have little or no impact on improving health outcomes" (*U.S. Federal Register*, 1989, p. 4309). It added that the provision would codify its authority *not* to cover a service viewed as marginally safe and effective, but expensive compared with available covered alternatives.

In the proposed regulations, HCFA defined cost-effectiveness and put forth the analytical steps it would follow, stating that they were "well accepted by economists." Specifically, HCFA said that cost-effectiveness would give the program authority to cover services in the following categories:

i. Very expensive to the program but provides significant benefits not otherwise available;
ii. Less costly and at least as effective as alternative covered intervention;
iii. More effective and more costly but added benefit justifies cost;
iv. Less effective and less costly but a viable alternative.

Finally, HCFA noted that it was aware that CEA was a complex field that suffered from data limitations and the inability to quantify some costs.

Aftermath of the 1989 proposed regulations. As a front-page *New York Times* story noted, the 1989 proposed regulations signaled a fundamental shift in U.S. health policy, giving Medicare the authority to weigh cost as a factor in reimbursing new technologies (Pear, 1991). Despite internal approval within the Department of Health and Human Services, however, the 1989 proposed regulations were never released in final form. Opposition came from the medical-device industry and from consumer groups such as the American Association of Retired Persons (AARP), who argued that the policy would lead to "rationing" (Pear, 1991).

HCFA's attempt in the mid-1990s to resurrect the cost-effectiveness provision and to publish the 1989 proposal regulation as a final rule met with stiff opposition. In a 1996 letter to the HCFA administrator, Bruce Vladeck, a broad-based group of medical and industry groups[4] opposed the idea, citing the passage of time since the 1989 regulation and the controversial nature of various elements, particularly the cost-effectiveness provision (American College of Physicians et al., 1996). The letter noted, for example, that "with respect to the cost-effectiveness issue, the U.S. Public Health Service has recently published a report titled 'Cost-Effectiveness in Health and Medicine,' which raises a number of significant questions with respect to the methodology associated with many cost-effectiveness analyses. . . . How HCFA plans to conduct cost-effectiveness analyses . . . is an issue that should be subject to the public comment process." The letter also stated that "Failure to seek and incorporate public comment may result in a rule that could inappropriately deprive Medicare beneficiaries of access to life-saving, life-enhancing medical technology."

Representative Bill Thomas, the chair of the powerful House Ways and Means committee, also opposed the plan to issue the regulation in final form (Ways & Means, 1997). At a congressional hearing in 1997, HCFA Administrator Vladeck acknowledged that:

> It is apparent that cost-effectiveness analysis is extremely controversial for beneficiaries, providers, and suppliers. It raises fears of rationing based on cost. HCFA has not and does not intend to make coverage decisions based solely on cost-effectiveness, and we will not refuse to cover services merely because they are costly. Moreover, manufacturers or providers do not need to submit formal cost-effectiveness analyses to HCFA in order to have a service considered for coverage (U.S. Congress, 1997).

MCAC and beyond. In 1999 HCFA formally announced that it was withdrawing its 1989 regulation (Federal Register, 1999).[5] By then, in response to persistent criticisms that its process needed to be more consistent, trans-

parent, and evidence-based, HCFA had established a new entity, the
Medicare Coverage Advisory Committee (MCAC), to advise the program
about the evidence of new medical technologies for coverage considerations
(Federal Register, 1998). The MCAC was created to counsel HCFA as to
whether specific medical items and services were reasonable and necessary under Medicare law using unbiased contemporary considerations of
"state-of-the-art" technology and science.

The MCAC helped HCFA shore up the evidence base for national
coverage decisions.[6] This was an important departure from the previous
policy, whereby the evidentiary basis was dictated by a standard of what
was "generally accepted in medical community" (Tunis and Kang, 2001).
Medicare officials have argued that since its creation, MCAC has helped
ensure a more consistent analytical framework, and wider participation—
not just of physicians, but also of methodologists, industry representatives,
and consumer advocates—as well as a more consistent, explicit, and open
process (Tunis and Kang, 2001). Unlike the previous process, for example,
the MCAC adheres to Federal Advisory Committee Act rules under which
meetings are open to the public, for example.

But a subsequent proposed Notice, which defined the criteria MCAC
would use in judging the "reasonable and necessary" clause made no
mention of cost-effectiveness (*U.S. Federal Register*, 2000). In the Notice,
MCAC assigned a very narrow role to cost, stating that it would consider
costs only in circumstances where a new service provided equivalent benefits to an existing Medicare-covered alternative and did not provide equivalent or lower costs (*U.S. Federal Register*, 2000; Garber, 2001). Even this
diluted Notice never released as a formal regulation. CMS still does not
want, or cannot afford politically for the program to be seen as an agent of
cost-containment rather than a vehicle to improve care (Garber, 2001). CMS
officials in recent years have again conceded that cost-effectiveness analysis has been "incredibly controversial." Former administrator Tom Scully
stated, "It's tough to say no to a cancer drug no matter how slender the
benefits" (Lagnado, 2003b).

Managed Care and Private Insurers

Given their incentives to deliver care efficiently, one might expect
managed-care plans to be among the most enthusiastic consumers of cost-
effectiveness information. Plans, however, have been reluctant to use the
technique openly.

Plans *have* used ever more aggressive and sophisticated processes for managing care, from utilization-review policies to disease-management programs. They have implemented "evidence-based" policies to avoid paying for ineffective care and to ensure that resources are targeted efficiently (Garber, 2001). To curtail rising drug costs, plans have employed a host of new policies, including charging higher co-payments for using expensive drugs, requiring prior approval before physicians can prescribe certain medications, calling physicians who prescribe more than recommended doses, profiling physicians to monitor high-cost prescribers, and even asking doctors in some cases to tell patients to switch to higher doses of drugs and then to break pills in half to save money (Kowalczyk, 2002).

But few, if any, plans are using cost-effectiveness as a formal policy tool. Neither scholarly overviews about managed-care practices (Gold, 1999) nor expansive press accounts about managed-care plan policies (Kowalczyk, 2002) mention explicit use of CEA. Similarly, reviews of the practices of pharmaceutical benefits managers (PBMs), the entities that administer and manage pharmaceutical benefits for health plans, health maintenance organizations (HMO)s, and employers, do not even bring up explicit use of CEA (Mathematica, 2000). Surveys of health plan officials about how they make coverage determinations reveal the importance decision makers place on factors such as FDA approval status, safety, effectiveness, the availability of alternative treatments in covering new health services, and the acquisition cost of the technology in question, but do not mention explicit cost-effectiveness analysis as a key input (e.g., Luce et al., 1996; Sloan et al., 1997; Titlow et al., 2000; Schoonmaker et al., 2000). Investigators emphasize the reluctance respondents report in wanting to discuss costs or cost-effectiveness with contracted providers or plan members (Singer and Bergthold, 2001).

Investigations into how managed-care officials make coverage decisions under budget constraints find no use of comparative cost-effectiveness analyses, despite intense competition among plans (Daniels and Sabin, 2002). Even in the few instances where medical directors mention CEA as an important component, it has not translated into explicit policy (e.g., Singer et al., 1999).

Health insurance contracts typically define covered services as those that are "medically reasonable and necessary" (Rosenbaum et al., 1999). Yet, seldom do definitions of medical necessity mention cost-effectiveness (Jacobson and Kanna, 2001; Sacremento Health Care Decisions, 2001). One large review of "medical necessity" language used in plans found that existing definitions of medical necessity fail to provide guidance to those who wish to make evidence-based decisions or explicitly make tradeoffs (Singer and Bergthold, 2001).

In excluding a service for coverage, health plans routinely appeal to the medical necessity clause, but rarely do they exclude services on grounds that they are not cost-effective. Plans also exclude services based on broad categories stated in private insurance contracts as ineligible for reimbursement—such as cosmetic services or unproven therapies—but again, these exclusions are based on medical rather than cost-effectiveness criteria (Garber, 2001).

The Blue Cross Blue Shield Technology Evaluation Center, which serves subscribing health plans and provider groups, has established an evidence-based process for determining whether to cover a new technology, but in the past has excluded explicit considerations of cost (Garber, 2001). Instead, the plan considers factors such as whether the technology has final approval from appropriate governmental bodies, whether scientific evidence permits conclusions concerning the effect of the technology on health outcomes, and whether the technology is as beneficial as any established alternative (Garber, 2001).

This development comes despite the growing power of insurers to make treatment decisions about what goods and services they will pay for. Escalating health costs have shifted control from physicians to insurers in reviewing decisions and dictating professional standards (Rosenbaum et al., 1999); however, it has not created any impetus for them to use CEA in their process.

In the few cases where CEA has been used explicitly, it has more than anything else proven the difficulty of doing so. One large health plan in the Midwest, which for years had promised in its mission statement to provide "exceptional quality, *cost-effective* care" (italics added) eventually removed the term "cost-effective" as objectionable (Jennifer Lafata, Henry Ford Health System, personal communication).[7]

Eddy (1992b) describes the uphill battle in the early 1990s to use cost-effectiveness as a guideline for decisions about the use of intravenous contrast agents in radiographic procedures in the Kaiser Permanente Southern California Region, a large group-practice health maintenance organization. First, plan officials agonized over whether they could prevail if sued because of the cost-effectiveness provision, and whether the non-financial cost of bad publicity would be worth the benefit of the improved decision. In the end, they decided that consideration of cost-effectiveness was reasonable, because the explicit nature of the decision was important to bring to light the implicit and anonymous process, because they were convinced that customers really wanted to control costs, and because they believed that they couldn't back off from tough decisions (Eddy, 1992b). Ultimately, however, their experience is the exception to the rule and illustrates above all the huge barriers to applying CEA in health policy-making.

Other Corners of U.S. Health-Care Policy

It is also difficult to find explicit use of CEA in other corners of U.S. health policy. One example involves the FDA's efforts to improve the safety of America's blood supply, after fears about HIV contamination arose in the 1980s (O'Grady, 2001). FDA shifted to ever more restrictive screening of blood donors by requiring additional testing for HIV and hepatitis B and C (HBV and HCV) among other measures.

The result has been undeniably safer blood but higher costs for the system due to the reduced donor pool and the increased costs of donor recruitment. The efforts have yielded small improvements in health relative to the increased costs. Researchers have estimated that the new U.S. policy translates to millions of dollars expended for each additional quality-adjusted life year gained, an estimate that far exceeds traditional standards for reasonableness (Aubuchon, 2000; Jackson et al., 2003), and which diverts funds from other more cost-effective improvements in health care and public health (O'Grady, 2001). The result has been increased blood prices for hospitals—though not increased Medicare payments. As one observer notes: "CMS's payments for blood have not kept up with the price increases resulting for the FDA's actions, but given the questionable cost-effectiveness of the FDA's actions, it is not clear CMS should be increasing payments" (O'Grady, 2001).[8]

Other examples abound. Clinical guidelines infrequently incorporate economic analyses. Few published guidelines mention economic analyses in their text or references, for example, even when high-quality economic evaluations are available (Wallace et al., 2002). Courts have not used CEA when instructing juries to consider evidence (Jacobson and Kanna, 2001). Studies show little relationship between the cost-effectiveness of public health and medical interventions and their actual implementation (Tengs and Graham, 1996) (Fig. 3–1). Surveys of physicians have shown that providing cost-effectiveness information tends to have little influence on their recommendations for familiar cervical, colon, and breast cancer screening (Ubel, Jepson et al., 2003). The key federal law governing Medicaid drug rebates, which imposes restrictions on the use of drug formularies, has lim-

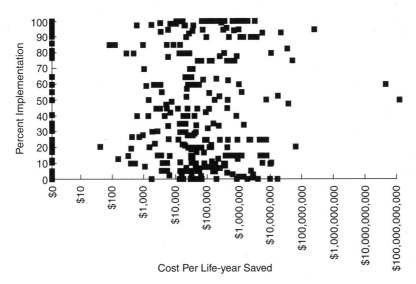

Figure 3–1. Costs of haphazard investments in life-saving. Implementation of life-saving interventions as a function of cost-effectiveness. *Source*: Tengs and Graham, 1996. Reproduced with permission.

ited state plans' ability to restrict drugs from coverage to clinical issues of safety and drug effectiveness, rather than cost-effectiveness (42 U.S.C. §1369r-8(d)(4)). The recently enacted Medicare drug benefit legislation authorizes the Agency for Health Care Research and Quality to conduct "comparative-effectiveness" not cost-effectiveness research, and even then states that the research cannot be used to withhold coverage of a prescription drug (Medicare Prescription Drug Improvement and Modernization Act, 2003).

4

Understanding the Resistance

. . . .

The man in the street is highly skeptical of the value of cost-effectiveness analysis: their unpopularity is scarcely surprising, if only because when beliefs conflict with evidence, beliefs tend to win.

—Drummond Rennie, 2001

One theory about resistance to cost-effectiveness analysis is that the technique has actually been used widely, but in ways that are difficult to detect or quantify. Perhaps it has even been influential in the United States, but quietly, under the radar. That possibility is considered in chapter 7. Even if true, however, the reluctance to use CEA as an explicit tool, at a time of soaring health spending and the widespread promotion of the technique to the medical community, warrants investigation.

In the last few years, a body of literature has accumulated around the attempt to understand decision makers' views about cost-effectiveness information and to explain their reluctance to use it. Reasons for their resistance generally fall into one of six categories: (1) lack of understanding, (2) mistrust of methods, (3) mistrust of motives, (4) legal and regulatory constraints, (5) political factors, and (6) ethical objections. This chapter considers the first three factors. The next chapter considers explanations (4) and (5) as well as a critique of cost-effectiveness analysis from medical ethicists and moral philosophers.

Lack of Understanding

A favorite explanation is that the decision makers simply fail to grasp the principles of CEA, that they are either ignorant or suffer from a kind of cost-effectiveness "innumeracy" when exposed to the information.

CEA is relatively new to medicine, and requires a kind of abstract thinking that many decision makers are not accustomed to (Eddy 1992a; Ubel, 2000). Some claim that physicians fundamentally don't understand—and haven't been taught—to think deeply about resource constraints and tradeoffs, or that their limited exposure has not provided them sufficient appreciation of economic concepts. Physicians misuse terminology and confuse concepts, not distinguishing between costs and cost-effectiveness, for example (Doubilet et al., 1986). They do not understand how to use decision-analytical methods or how to apply concepts such as incremental cost-effectiveness ratios or quality-adjusted life years (Ginsberg et al., 2000). Doctors confuse average and incremental cost-effectiveness ratios (Hershey et al., 2003). They don't appreciate the value of models to explore alternative clinical scenarios or the uncertainty of parameter estimates (Eddy, 1992a; Duthie et al., 1999; Prosser, 2000).

Results of CEAs can be counterintuitive, especially to clinicians used to thinking about the importance of a service in terms of its relative effectiveness rather than its cost-effectiveness, and used to thinking about clinical problems from the individual patient's rather than the populations' perspective (Eddy, 1992a). Doctors complain that CEAs make excessive use of assumptions rather than actual data (Drummond and Sculpher, 2003).

Clinicians' desire for simpler endpoints and disaggregated results, rather than cost-effectiveness ratios, has also been cited. It has been argued, for example, that using cost-utility analysis to study interventions that affect only quality of life rather than length of life (e.g., sildenafil [Viagra]) is misleading (McGregor, 2003). The Panel on Cost-Effectiveness itself notes that "CEA can be used to evaluate interventions for treating schizophrenia and for treating heart disease. But the health outcomes are so different that it is difficult to capture them in the same measurement system and direct comparisons of the QALYs created by the two kinds of interventions may not yet be possible" (Gold et al., p. 12, cited in McGregor, 2003). Surveys of health decision makers corroborate these attitudes, confirming a lack of expertise and a misunderstanding of economic concepts as key problems for decision makers in the United States and abroad (Zellmer, 1995; Sloan et al., 1997; Duthie, 1999; Stoykova et al., 2000; Grizzle et al., 2000; Annell and Svarvar, 2000).

A related complaint is about the perceived lack of transparency in CEA—that analyses are incomprehensible "black boxes" and that the process obscures important value judgments inherent in them (Heinzerling and Ackerman, 2002). In David Eddy's imaginary conversation with his father, Maxon Eddy says that the language of mathematics is foreign to most practitioners: "clinicians feel left out or put down by people conducting analyses . . . they can't check the calculations to make sure it is being done right. . . ." (Eddy 1992a). Critics complain that the highly complex, expert-driven nature of economic evaluation makes it extremely difficult for the public to understand and participate (Heinzerling and Ackerman, 2002).

Policy makers, too, have questioned the abstract nature of CEAs. In a hearing on Medicare coverage policy before the House of Representatives Ways and Means Committee in 1997 (U.S. Congress, 1997), Committee Chairman Representative Thomas (R-CA) said: "if [the intervention] is going to reduce the long-term morbidity for diabetics, we ought to do it and we should not get caught up in some of the very arcane theoretical cost-effectiveness arguments at all." At another point in the hearing, he said, "we are currently facing a discussion with the Congressional Budget Office on the cost-effectiveness of a number of preventive procedures and they persist in indicating to us that there is a cost associated with these, and we are trying to explain to them: No, it saves money" (U.S. Congress, 1997). Later, Thomas questioned the concepts of discounting and quality-of-life adjustments.[1]

While illuminating some measure of the resistance, however, lack of understanding falls short as an explanation. For one thing, complaints about conceptual misunderstandings go back a long way (e.g., Eddy 1992a): more progress might have been expected by now. For another, clinicians routinely incorporate abstract concepts—on statistics, or genetics, or the acid-based balance—into their decisions (Eddy, 1992a).

More important, the rationale doesn't explain the resistance of *policy makers*. Given their incentives to allocate resources more efficiently, policy makers should reasonably be expected to educate themselves or contract out for assistance, as they have in other instances. Medicare has implemented numerous complex programs, from prospective payment systems to the resource-based relative value scale. Managed care has employed sophisticated tools of utilization review. Policy makers' failure to adopt CEA suggests less a lack of understanding than a kind of willful neglect.

Mistrust of Methods

A second explanation points to a lack of trust in the methods, rather than a lack of understanding per se. CEA, it is said, suffers from a credibility problem, which stems from various sources, including methodological discrepancies across analyses, a lack of standards for the field, and a perception that even well-conducted studies are not relevant to the practical needs of decision makers.

Methodological discrepancies/absence of standards

At the outset of its book, the Panel on Cost-Effectiveness comments that "lack of a common set of techniques in cost-effectiveness analysis has restrained the applicability of studies in policy context" (Gold et al., 1996, p. vii). Indeed, the Panel's *raison d'être* relates to the need for methodological consistency: "valid comparisons of cost-effectiveness ratios across studies require that the numerators and denominators be reported in similar terms and be obtained using comparable methods."

Researchers have long known that the CEA methods used differ from study to study, and that adherence to recommended protocols is often, even generally, lacking (see, for example, Udvarhelyi et al., 1992; Gerard, 1992; Adams et al., 1992; Birch and Gafni, 1994; Mason et al., 1993; Brown and Fintor, 1993; Nord, 1993; Briggs and Sculpher, 1995; Blackmore and Magid, 1997; Neumann et al., 1997; Balas et al., 1998; Jefferson et al., 1998; Graham et al., 1998; Gerard et al., 1999; Neumann et al., 2000; Chapman et al., 2000; Stone et al., 2000; Bell et al., 2000; Jefferson et al., 2002).

Published cost-effectiveness analyses have differed in the ways they have conceptualized and estimated costs (Dranove, 1995; Balas et al., 1998; Stone et al., 2000) and quality-adjusted life years gained (Nord, 1993; Neumann et al., 1997; Chapman et al., 2000; Neumann et al., 2000c; Bell et al., 2000; Adam et al., 2003). Studies have varied considerably in their inclusion of overhead costs, inclusion of indirect costs due to illness or informal care or volunteer time; and inclusion of health-care costs for unrelated illness in added years of life (Adam et al., 2003). They have also differed in the methods used to convert foreign currencies to U.S. dollars (i.e., whether they use foreign-exchange rates or purchasing power parity (Adam et al., 2003).

Published CEAs also vary with respect to factors such as the perspective assumed in the analysis, the discount rate used to adjust for future costs and benefits, and how uncertainty is defined (Udvarhelyi et al., 1992; Briggs and Sculpher, 1995; Neumann et al., 2000a; Chapman et al., 2000; Petrou et al., 2000; Drummond and Sculpher, 2003). Other methodological flaws include incorrectly characterizing the comparator intervention or inappropriately extrapolating beyond the period observed in the clinical study (Drummond and Sculpher, 2003).

Many published CEAs fail to provide a clear description of methods, or lack explanation and justification of the framework and approach they use. Others have poor estimates for the effectiveness of the interventions they evaluate, selectively report results, or mischaracterize the overall findings of the analysis (Azimi and Welch, 1998; Chapman et al., 2000; Neumann et al., 2000; Jefferson et al., 2002; Drummond and Sculpher, 2003). Some analyses report cost-effectiveness ratios on an average rather than incremental basis (Chapman et al., 2000; Drummond and Sculpher, 2003), which can mask the high price for achieving incremental health-care goals (Hershey et al., 2003).

Evaluations of the same interventions using different methods can lead to very different results (Brown and Fintor, 1993). Even well-conducted CEAs of the same strategy can come to different conclusions. Pignone and colleagues (2002) recently reviewed seven high-quality CEAs on colorectal cancer screening, each of which met all of the authors' strict inclusion/exclusion criteria. While all came to the conclusion that screening was relatively cost-effective compared to no screening (with C/E ratios between $10,000 and $25,000 per life year [in $U.S. 2000]), no particular screening strategy was consistently found to be the most cost-effective. Studies differed on dimensions, such as assumptions about the biological behavior of colorectal cancer, screening adherence, complications of colonoscopy, the costs considered, and the type of strategy considered (e.g., the age at which screening should be stopped).

Methodological differences and poor-quality studies appear both in the peer-reviewed literature and in CEAs submitted to reimbursement authorities.[2] Hill et al. (2000), for example, reported significant problems in pharmacoeconomic analyses submitted to the Australian Pharmaceutical Benefits Scheme from 1994 through 1997: of 326 submissions, 218 (67%) had serious problems of interpretation—particularly with the degree of uncertainty in estimates of comparative clinical efficacy, modeling issues, cost estimates, and the choice of comparator. A study of 95 submissions to the Canadian Coordinating Office of Health Technology Assessment (CCOHTA) between 1996 and 1999 found that a high percentage had missing information and inappropriate data (e.g., use of inappropriate comparator or time horizon) (Anis and Gagnon, 2000). An analysis of submissions to the Comitato Interna-Ministeriale Programmazione Economica of the Italian Ministry of Health—the body responsible for national drug-reimbursement negotiations in Italy—reported recurring problems of pharmacoeconomic analyses based on unproven differences in effectiveness and questions about utility assessments (Messori et al., 2000). Atherly et al. (2001) evaluated the scope and content of 50 dossiers of evidence submitted by drug companies to the Regence health plan in Seattle from January 1998 to June 2000, and found that many dossiers were incomplete in their inclusion of economic models, budget impact analyses, and other economic information.

Moreover, the argument goes cost-effectiveness researchers continue to debate certain fundamental questions, such as which costs to include in the numerator of the cost-effectiveness ratio (i.e., whether costs associated with lost ability to work should be included, or whether loss of productivity due to death is implicitly incorporated in the QALY calculation) (Brouwer et al., 1998; Meltzer and Johannesson, 1999; Garber, 1999; Russell, 1999; Weinstein, 1999).

Similar debates continue over which techniques and whose preferences to use in QALY calculations.[3] It has long been known that different utility-elicitation methods (for example, the standard gamble versus time-tradeoff approach) yield different estimates (Read et al., 1984; Hornberger et al., 1992; Nease et al., 1995; O'Leary et al., 1995; Bleichrodt and Johannesson, 1996; Nord, 1996; Van Wijck et al., 1998; Glick et al., 1999). Researchers have used estimates for the disutility due to impotence ranging from 0.26 to 0.02, for example (McGregor, 2003); estimates for the utilities associated with liver cancer have ranged from 0.1 to 0.49 (Bell et al., 2001).[4]

Individual preferences may be inconsistent with the strict assumptions of expected utility theory that underlie the QALY concept, such as the assumption of constant proportional tradeoffs between longevity and quality of life (which holds that one would be willing to give up some fraction of one's life years in order to improve the quality of those years from one level to a preferred level, and that the fraction depends only on the two quality levels and not on the length of life at the outset).[5]

The discrepancies and lack of rigor have contributed to a lingering sense that the methodology is not ready for prime time (Kassirer and Angell, 1994; Evans, 1995; Rennie and Luft, 2000; Rennie, 2001). CEAs are considered malleable. Maxon Eddy wonders aloud if CEA is solid enough for real decisions (Eddy 1992c): if one cannot reliably make comparisons across cost-effectiveness ratios, he wonders, then why use the approach to inform policy?

The movement in the medical community towards evidence-based medicine seems, if anything, to have intensified the concern of some observers about cost-effectiveness analysis. It has strengthened faith in randomized controlled trials and in observed data over the projections from models that are used typically in CEAs. It has provided further ammunition to physicians and policy makers who were already skeptical about the assumptions and extrapolations of cost-effectiveness analyses.

Methodological discrepancies, while real, do not explain CEA's plight, however. Despite incongruities between studies, a broad consensus has long existed over the basic components and protocols that *should* compose well-conducted and reported CEAs. This encompasses the need for clarity in framing and reporting analyses, including full disclosure of all funding sources and adhering to basic tenets for presenting study assumptions and basic information about costs and preference weights (Weinstein and Stason, 1977; Drummond et al., 1987).

This harmony is reflected in the similarity among national guidelines for using CEA as part of the decision-making process for new drugs and other technologies.[6] The guidelines share many features in terms of methodological and reporting requirements, such as the analysis framework and the types of costs and health outcomes to be estimated and reported; the format for modeling, time horizon, discounting, sensitivity analyses, and the presentation of results; and the inclusion of "financial impact" or "budget impact" analyses. The differences that do exist between the guidelines—the choice of perspective, or whether "indirect" costs should be included—are relatively minor and easily disclosed (Drummond, 1999; Hjelmgren et al., 2001).

Moreover, some peer-reviewed journals have adopted guidelines and checklists for authors, referees, and editors in order to improve editorial management and the quality of manuscripts (Drummond et al., 1996), or have required structured abstracts for CEAs to improve reporting (Mittmann et al., 1998, Rosen et al., 2003). Though there is still much room for improvement, the quality of published CEAs has improved over time, especially in top-tier journals (Neumann et al., 2000; Jefferson et al., 2002). Since publication of the report of the Panel on Cost-Effectiveness Analysis, more analyses are adhering to recommended protocols (Phillips and Chen, 2002).

Lack of relevance

Another aspect of the problem is a perceived lack of relevance. Policy analysts have often commented on the disconnection between the abstract, academic ideal of CEAs and the working needs of actual decision makers, particularly those in managed-care plans. Even advocates of CEA have acknowledged that barriers concerning relevance are at least as important as those related to methods (Prosser et al., 2000).

CEAs typically do not explore budget impacts. Decision makers find savings claimed in analyses illusory (Langley, 2000). They complain that the C/E ratio, reported as costs per life-years gained or costs per QALYs gained, is unhelpful, if not irrelevant, to decision makers, who worry day-to-day about short-term financial shortfalls and budgetary "silos" rather than the long-term horizon and societal perspective called for by academics

(Berger, 1999). Health plans, some say, are not in the business of purchasing QALYs.

Health insurers—and employers—are concerned about *affordability*, which depends on the overall volume of patients and is typically ignored in analyses (Drummond, 2002). Payers believe that they can get into financial difficulty by adopting too many cost-effective interventions, just as families can bankrupt themselves by purchasing too many bargain-price items (Drummond et al., 2002; Ubel, Hirth et al., 2003). Conversely, payers may be willing to adopt an intervention with an unfavorable C/E ratio if it affects a small number of people, especially if this helps avoid adverse publicity and has a minor effect on the bottom line. Simple rankings of C/E ratios can thus mask important differences across studies—in the magnitude of benefit, or in the uncertainty of estimates.

Langley (2000) argues that rather than blame managed-care decision makers for failing to understand CEAs, the field needs to accept that "the methodology that characterizes the majority of cost-effectiveness analysis is simply not relevant to a managed care audience—or indeed to any other health system audience." He claims that traditional CEA is too narrow, and its assumptions are highly unrealistic. It doesn't capture the complexity of patients, and doesn't anticipate the practical information needs of formulary decision makers. Langley concludes that the approach simply isn't useful as a tool for managing budgets. Managers, he argues, need to know how use of a service affects the plans' own outcome profiles and costs.

Cost-effectiveness analysts often ignore considerations of generalizability (Murray et al., 2000; Drummond and Sculpher, 2003; Hutubessy et al., 2002). Analysts often ask the wrong questions, focusing narrowly on drugs or individual procedures rather than broader strategies like quality initiatives or disease-management programs (Neumann et al, 2003). Moreover, given the sizeable resources required to conduct CEAs, only a fraction of the possible strategies are ever considered formally, raising questions about the relevance of studies that are conducted.

Among published CEAs, the C/E ratio in one setting or health-care system may be irrelevant to another (Litvak et al., 2000). Results of CEAs are highly context-specific and cannot inform policy debates in another population or setting (Murray et al., 2000). As Hutubessy et al. (2002) point out, in practice many factors affect cost-effectiveness: the availability of an intervention, the mix and quality of inputs, local prices, implementation capacity, underlying organizational structures and incentives, and supporting institutional framework.

Analyses typically neglect practical issues concerning the implementation of the service in question. Litvak et al. (2000) point out that an analysis may show surgery to be more cost-effective than medications, but rarely if ever do investigators account for the increased demand for surgery that may result if the plan adopts the strategy—and attending problems it may cause such as increasing waiting times for operating rooms, which in turn can ripple through the hospital. Analysts assume incorrectly that resources can be easily redirected (Murray et al., 2000). Hutubessy et al. (2002) note that changing from cost-ineffective to cost-effective strategies incurs transactions costs that are typically neglected in cost-effectiveness analyses.

Murray et al. (2000) argue that existing cost-effectiveness analyses do not allow an examination of whether current practice is efficient and should have been done in first place. In their view incremental analysis may not be relevant for many decision makers because the starting point for analyses varies across settings (according to current state of infrastructure and current mix of interventions). Moreover, the additional health effectiveness achieved from a given increase in resource use depends on the current level of spending (Murray et al., 2000). They note that the cost and effectiveness of delivering antimalarial drugs closer to households will depend critically on whether a network of village workers currently exists or on current and past environmental management of malarial control (Hutubessy et al., 2002). More generally, analysts typically ignore non-linear cost-effectiveness functions: i.e., the cost per QALY of expanding a program from 30% to 40% is likely to be much lower than cost per QALY through expansion of coverage from 80% to 90% (Murray et al., 2000).

Surveys of health officials reflect these concerns. They underscore the relative unimportance of CEAs compared with factors such as clinical evidence, risks and harms of therapy, the availability of alternative treatments, and the existence of authoritative guidelines or generally accepted standards (e.g., Luce et al., 1996; Titlow et al., 2000; Ubel et al., 2003). When asked specifically about cost-effectiveness information, decision makers say they want simpler, more targeted, and more timely information, more germane to their own decisions or guidelines (Steiner et al., 1996; Sloan et al., 1997; Drummond, 1997; Duthie et al., 1999; Grizzle et al., 2000; Annell and Svarvar, 2000; Stoykova et al., 2000; Crump, 2000; Hoffman et al., 2002).

The CEA establishment has been curiously reticent on the matter. *The Panel on Cost-Effectiveness* does not contain any mention of "budget impact" analyses, for example. To the extent it deals with the question of CEA's relevance, it does so obliquely, in theoretical discussions about which "perspective" an analysis should take.

The actual perspective assumed in a CEA can matter greatly. A drug may be cost-effective from the payer's perspective, but not from society's, for example. From the societal perspective, drugs for Alzheimer's disease may reduce some nursing home costs but at the expense of unpaid caregivers. No single health plan or government payer actually incurs caregiving costs, yet they loom large in the burden of Alzheimer's disease and the cost-effectiveness of treatment (see Neumann et al., 1999; O'Brien et al., 1999).

The Panel discusses perspective at some length (Gold et al., pp. 185–7; 289–290). However, beyond recommending that analysts conduct CEAs from multiple perspectives in secondary analyses in order to satisfy the demands of individual decision makers (Gold et al., p. 185), the discussion sidesteps the broader ideological question it begs: how health-care markets should work.

Advocating the societal perspective made eminent sense for the Panel, given its wide mandate to consider tools for allocating societal resources— and its funding from the U.S. Public Health Service. But advocating the reference case also assumed a world-view that exposed a rift between the ideals of the public health community and the practical demands of private plans, and added fuel to the firestorm over "relevance."

The lack of a single payer in the United States creates an inherent problem for the application of CEA. No individual payer in the United States actually assumes the societal perspective. Private insurers, which cover most of the U.S. population, have truncated time horizons. While private plans do respond to enrollee and employer demands and compete with other plans in the marketplace, all of which provides incentives to deliver high-quality care, they tend not to consider the societal perspective. Plans experience rapid enrollee turnover. They do not pay for long-term care and certain other health-care services. They do not incur costs for lost productivity or for patient travel and time.

Application of tools like CEA makes the most sense in the absence of well-functioning markets, which means that private-sector resource allocation tools—capital budgeting or return on investment—are insufficient (Warner and Luce, 1982). CEAs (and CBAs) in health care have found the widest acceptance in pure public goods in which certain conditions hold: provision to one individual benefits all individuals; no one can be excluded from receiving the benefits; and one person's consumption of a benefit does not reduce its availability. Thus, the original applications to water-resource management projects (Warner and Luce, 1982). CEA raises peculiar difficulties when applied to private health-care consumption because the social benefits are difficult to quantify and value (Fein, 1976; Warner and Luce, 1982).

Still, one can make a good argument that at the very least a program such as Medicare should use CEA and assume a societal perspective, given that it is a broad social program financed largely from general tax revenues or payroll taxes. Medicare's failure to do so may reflect the fact that public officials respond to the narrow incentives they confront even when administering social programs. Medicare does not cover certain health costs such as long-term care or (until recently) outpatient prescription drugs. This limits Medicare's incentives to use CEAs from the societal perspective.

In the end, "lack of relevance" also falls short as an explanation. Why haven't payers like Medicare or Medicaid simply funded or conducted their own analyses and tailored them to their needs as they have in other countries? The real answer to the question about why policy makers in the United States have failed to use CEA seems to lay elsewhere—in the lack of trust people have in the analysts conducting CEAs, or in legal or regulatory constraints, or perhaps because CEAs, even when well done, do not reflect how society really wants to allocate its health resources. I turn to these possibilities next.

Mistrust of Motives

A more cynical explanation for the resistance to CEA questions not the methods per se, but the *motives* of investigators and their sponsors. A perception prevails that analyses reflect the biases of investigators with a financial stake in the outcomes. Curiously this account has roots in two very different sources.

On one hand, CEA is seen as a smokescreen for cost-cutting efforts. Physicians and the public may view CEA as an accounting or cost-management tool, or that it is a code word for rationing. Clinicians suspect health-plan managers of using CEA to intrude on their sovereignty in order to improve the bottom line (Ubel, 2000; Jacobson and Kanna, 2001). Their frustration with CEA reflects in part a territorial issue and a fear of losing control (Eddy 1992a). Surveys of physicians suggest that their unwillingness to use CEA may relate to their belief that any money saved will go into the salaries of insurance company executives and the profits of insurance company owners, rather than to improve the health of the population (Asch et al., 2003).

The other strain of mistrust radiates from a different direction: CEA is perceived as a tool that those with a financial gain at stake can use to *increase* health expenditure.

Studies support the tendency of cost-effectiveness analysts to conclude that additional expenditures are warranted for the service under investigation (Azimi and Welch, 1998; Neumann et al., 2000). Few investigators, regardless of their backgrounds or sources of funding, report unfavorable cost-effectiveness ratios (Azimi and Welch, 1998; Neumann et al., 2000).[7] Brown (1991) has noted that "cost-effectiveness enables programs that can credibly wear its mantle to stand out from the crowd. But ... its impact has been largely asymmetrical: useful in justifying the expansion of programs, but seldom significant in eliminating services." Studies find that to the extent that clinical guidelines incorporate CEAs, they do so by incorporating favorable ratios (Ramsey, 2002).

Although using CEA to champion an intervention may be widespread, critics have focused their attacks on studies sponsored by the pharmaceutical industry. Critics of industry-funded CEAs have long complained that CEAs reflect the hidden biases of industry sponsors and that the field owes more to marketers than to scientists (e.g., Kassirer and Angell, 1994; Evans, 1995). Rennie (2001) has written that cost-effectiveness analyses funded by drug companies rarely reach unfavorable conclusions, that good methods are flouted, and that marketers often choose ineffective comparison drugs, pull unsympathetic researchers off studies, block publication, or control data.

Over the years, the pharmaceutical industry has increasingly colonized the field of economic evaluation (though government funding remains an important source, especially for cost-utility analyses). Of 228 CUAs published between 1976 and 1997, for example, 54% were sponsored by government organizations or foundations, and 14% by pharmaceutical and device companies; Of 294 CUAs published between 1998 and 2001, the proportion of government/foundation sponsored studies fell to 43%, while drug company–funded studies increased to 20% (in each time period about one third of the authors did not disclose the funding source) (Fig. 4–1).

Almost all large drug (and medical device) companies, and many smaller ones, have formalized the performance and support of cost-effectiveness analyses—often called *health economics* or *outcomes research*—within their firms (DiMasi et al., 2001). By 2000, departments in charge of the function typically had budgets of $5–$20 million, with 15–20 full-time equivalents (FTEs), and they contracted out about half of their work as well (DiMasi et al.,

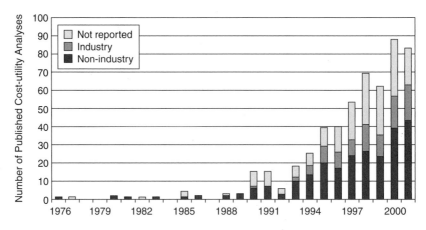

Figure 4–1.   Trends in sponsorship of cost-utility analyses, 1976–2001. *Source*: CEA registry, Harvard School of Public Health, 2003 (www.hsph.harvard/edu.cearegistry).

2001). A study by DiMasi et al. (2001) found that drug company officials expected the function to grow, with firms increasingly initiating pharmacoeconomic analyses early in clinical development and incorporating them into clinical trial design (DiMasi et al., 2001).

The pharmaceutical industry has rushed into the field for two reasons. In part, the trend reflects defensive posturing: as health plans gained market share in the 1990s, they began demanding (and in a few cases requiring) evidence that the increasingly expensive prescription drugs they were being asked to pay for offered demonstrated value. The pharmaceutical industry was left with no choice but to fund the analyses to provide the evidence. On the other hand, drug companies have also actively embraced pharmacoeconomics as a new opportunity to market their products on the basis of value and economic advantages.

Regardless of the reason, the trend clearly has cast suspicion on the field. Virtually all surveys of health decision makers reveal concerns about "biased" CEAs attributable to industry financing (Lax and Moench, 1995; Sloan et al., 1997; Drummond et al., 1997b; Grizzle et al., 2000; Motheral et al., 2000; Annell and Svarvar, 2000). Decision makers consistently cite "lack of credibility" as one of the greatest barriers to using CEA. Fewer than 20% of respondents in one survey agreed with the statement that "the comparative pharmacoeconomic claims made by drug manufacturers generally meet high standards for reliability" (Zellmer, 1995). Respondents also agree that a key part of making CEAs more useful lies in sponsoring more independent research and in ensuring objective external reviewers (e.g., Sloan et al., 1997).

The mistrust in industry-sponsored CEAs can be seen in the growing calls during the 1990s for better peer review of the field (e.g., Jefferson and Demicheli, 1995) and for stricter policies governing disclosure of conflicts-of-interest and of publication arrangements, such as requiring that authors retain the freedom to publish results without regard to the direction of the conclusions (Hillman et al., 1991; Schulman et al., 1994; Task Force on Principles, 1995).

The *New England Journal of Medicine* went so far as to issue a strongly worded policy statement imposing restrictions for publishing CEAs in its pages (Kassirer and Angell, 1994). The journal's editors said that they *would* consider high-quality CEAs, including those supported by industry. But manuscripts would have to meet certain conditions to warrant consideration: (1) industry-funded research must be in the form of a grant to a not-for-profit entity—there would be no review if the author received a direct salary or had an equity interest in the company, or was a member of an ongoing consultancy or board; (2) there must be assurances of authors' independence regarding issues of design, interpretation, publication, and access to data; and (3) manuscripts must include information about all data used and assumptions made, and the model must be straightforward and lucid.

Though other journals did not follow suit in disallowing authors who received industry funding directly, they did stiffen disclosure requirements, require authorial independence, tighten peer review, and publish guidelines for the content of economic studies (Drummond et al., 1996; Elstein, 1997; O'Brien et al., 1997).

How much influence does industry sponsorship actually have over CEA results? Several studies have reported that industry-funded CEAs are more likely than non–industry-sponsored research to report favorable findings (Azimi and Welch, 1998; Friedberg et al., 1999; Neumann et al., 2000b).

Precisely why this occurs is less clear. It could reflect a "publication bias" that may exist on several levels: drug company sponsors may only fund studies of products likely to show cost-effectiveness, or they may selectively bring to market drugs that provide good value (Neumann, 1998; Rennie and Luft, 2000; Gagnon, 2000). A more cynical explanation holds that sponsors may influence investigators to make favorable assumptions, or may restrict investigators from publishing negative results. Even without overt influence, investigators may be more inclined to submit analyses with favorable results for publication, and editors may selectively publish positive studies (King, 1996; Rennie, 1997).

The more interesting question is not why suspicions exist, but why heightened scrutiny is given CEAs compared with other areas of medical research.

After all, publication bias is a well-documented problem in the medical literature. Researchers have demonstrated that peer-reviewed journals are generally likelier to publish analyses with interesting or contentious findings, and less likely to publish negative or unfavorable results (Begg, 1994; Freemantle and Mason, 1997).

Moreover, many researchers have highlighted the influence of industry over clinical research (e.g., Blumenthal et al., 1986; Schwarz, 1991; Thompson, 1993; Lemmens and Singer, 1998; Krimsky and Rothenberg, 1998). Researchers have found that industry-sponsored drug trials rarely report that the drug under investigation is inferior to its comparator, and that there is a strong relationship between expert authors' published positions on the safety of some drugs and their financial relationships with pharmaceutical manufacturers (Rochon et al., 1994; Koepp and Miles, 1999; Stelfox, 1998).

But journals have not banned industry-affiliated authors of clinical trials from their pages (though they have attempted to enforce policies to disclose conflicts of interest). Nor have surveys detected the same levels of concern about other areas of medicine that decision makers have expressed about CEAs. Furthermore, studies have not detected evidence that the quality of CEAs funded by the industry differs from those funded by other sources (Neumann et al., 2000b).[8]

The reason for the discrepancy probably involves physicians' unfamiliarity with CEAs as well as the technique's heavy reliance on assumptions. Physicians trained in experimental methods view CEAs as reviews, which are more easily manipulated than are clinical trials (Kassirer and Angell, 1994). Relatively few published CEAs are conducted alongside randomized controlled trials (Greenberg et al., 2004). Rennie and Luft (2000) highlight several areas of concern: the lack of head-to-head trials upon which to base assumptions about effectiveness, the use of short-term surrogate markers to project long-term results, and the potential for analysts to selectively use cost and outcome data. In their *New England Journal of Medicine* editorial on CEAs, Kassirer and Angell (1994) commented: "We recognize that bias can compromise even original scientific studies, but we believe that the opportunities for introducing bias into economic studies are far greater, given the discretionary nature of model building, and data selection in the analysis. In addition, unlike the effectiveness side of the equation, which is based on biological phenomena, the cost side is highly artificial. Drug costs, in particular, can be quite arbitrary. . . ."

While mistrust of motives is a genuine factor in explaining opposition to CEA, it, too, falls short as a sufficient explanation. It does not explain why

institutional arrangements have not evolved to ensure investigator independence, for example. Nor does it clarify why the United States, unlike other
countries, has not enacted policies that rely on CEAs while avoiding or at
least reducing suspicions. In the next chapter, I turn to another possible
explanation, separate from the issue of trust: namely, that legal, regulatory,
and political barriers in the United States are to blame for CEA's troubles.

5

Legal, Political, and Ethical Concerns

. . . .

Perhaps statutory and regulatory factors explain why policy makers in the United States resist formal use of CEA. Federal or state laws may preclude its use, for example. Language written into private contracts may prevent it. Possibly, American proclivities to sue—and health providers' fears about how courts would view the use of CEA—present *de facto* barriers.

Medicare's Statutory Language as a Barrier

As noted in chapter 3, Medicare's authorizing legislation states that "No payment may be made for any expenses incurred for items and services that are not reasonable and necessary for the diagnosis or treatment of illness or injury" (1862(a)(1)(A) of the Social Security Act). When Medicare proposed in 1989 that it would use cost-effectiveness as a criterion in covering new technologies, it affirmed that its authority to do so stemmed from this key statutory clause—though, importantly, HCFA officials also believed that formal rule-making was prudent for this statement of interpretation (*U.S. Federal Register*, 1989).

As discussed, the 1989 proposed regulation was never published in final form. Moreover, subsequent attempts to interpret the "reasonable and necessary" clause make no mention of cost-effectiveness analysis (*U.S. Federal Register*, 2000).

But Medicare's failure to incorporate CEA was caused by political pressures rather than a lack of statutory or regulatory authority per se. A full policy and legal debate on whether the "reasonable and necessary" language imparts to Medicare the authority to use CEA has never taken place. Nevertheless, the 1989 proposed regulation, as well as attempts to revise the cost-effectiveness debate in the 1990s, signaled top Medicare officials' belief that the existing statute provided sufficient cover. While courts have not ruled on Medicare and cost-effectiveness per se, there is good reason to believe that courts would defer to the government's position on the matter, as long as the policy was not handled in an arbitrary or capricious manner (Jacobson and Kanna, 2001).

The FDA as a Barrier to the Dissemination of Cost-Effectiveness Information

In theory FDA rules could have some chilling effect on the production and use of cost-effectiveness analyses. The regulatory agency has traditionally concerned itself with matters of safety and efficacy rather than economics when deciding whether a drug warrants approval for the marketplace. The Agency, however, has long held authority to ensure that information disseminated by drug manufacturers is not inaccurate or misleading (Kessler and Pines, 1990). The emergence in the 1990s of drug companies' interest in promoting the economic advantages of their products confronted the FDA with a new dilemma: how to regulate promotional materials containing claims about a drug's "cost-effectiveness."

In 1995, the FDA's Division of Drug Marketing and Communications (DDMAC) issued draft guidelines on the issue, stipulating that health economic studies would be required to provide "substantial evidence typically demonstrated by two adequate and well-controlled studies" (U.S. FDA, 1995). The draft guidelines were criticized by some in the pharmaceutical industry and elsewhere on grounds that they favored randomized controlled trials (RCTs) for economic endpoints at the expense of "modeling" exercises, which lie at the heart of most cost-effectiveness analyses, and that they didn't appreciate the needs and growing sophistication of managed-care plans (Neumann et al., 1996).[1] The FDA's policy, critics rightfully argued, could impede the flow and use of cost-effectiveness information.

The 1997 Food and Drug Administration Modernization Act (FDAMA) codified rules about the evidentiary basis drug manufacturers needed to support economic claims about their products, and attempted to provide some additional flexibility for companies to make cost-effectiveness claims (FDAMA, P.L. 105–115; Neumann et al., 2000c).[2] Section 114 of the Act states that health care economic information (HCEI) disseminated by a manufacturer to a formulary committee or managed-care plan will not be considered false or misleading as long as it is based on "competent and reliable scientific evidence" and is "directly related to an approved indication" (FDAMA, P.L. 105–115).

In enacting Section 114, Congress sought at once to add flexibility to rules governing the exchange of health economic information and to carefully restrict the boundaries (Neumann et al., 2000c). By including the clause "directly related to an approved indication," Congress seriously circumscribed the ability of firms to make economic claims using Section 114, because—according to the Committee report that accompanied the legislation—"directly related" typically means substantiated by adequate and well-controlled trials (U.S. Congress, 1997).

For example, the manufacturer of a drug approved to treat symptoms of heart failure, but not to prolong survival, could not make an economic claim tied to extending survival (e.g., a cost/QALY estimate). The Committee report provides the example of a drug approved to alter bone mass density but not to affect hip fracture; an economic claim based on hip fracture prevention would not be permitted—even if observational data established a strong link from the surrogate marker (bone mass density) to the long-term endpoint (hip fracture prevention).

The "directly related" restriction prohibits manufacturers from using common forms of economic evaluation, such as cost-effectiveness and cost-utility analysis, to the extent that analyses use surrogate clinical endpoints to project long-term health outcomes, such as quality-adjusted survival. Notably, the rules would prohibit the promotion of reference case CEAs, despite the fact that the committee report stated that methods underlying HCEI would be assessed using standards "widely accepted by experts" (U.S. Congress, 1997; Neumann et al., 2000c).

What *is* permitted under these rules is less clear. Presumably, Section 114 allows claims that contain "costing studies," which simply assign monetary values to outcomes investigated in well-controlled trials. For example, if a randomized controlled trial demonstrates that Drug X reduces hospitalizations, manufacturers could estimate the net dollar savings involved and make an economic claim based on the results. As of mid 2004, FDA still had not provided any written guidance about Section 114 and seemed content to wait for marketplace reaction (Merrill, 1999; Neumann et al., 2000c).

These rules may also have impeded some exchange of cost-effectiveness information between drug manufacturers and their customers. But it is unlikely that it has provided a major or even a minor barrier to the use of CEA in the United States.

For one thing, companies have continued to promote messages about the economic advantages of their products in print advertisements and other media (Neumann et al., 2002; Stewart and Neumann, 2002). More important, the existence of Section 114 does not prevent health plans and government payers from *requesting* CEA information. Such demands would constitute "unsolicited requests" and thus sidestep FDA's evidentiary standards for promotional claims, as long as requests are truly unprompted and specific in nature (Neumann, 2004a). Such requests for economic data, particularly from drug formulary committees, are becoming more common, and greatly diminish the importance of Section 114, as discussed at greater length in chapter 7.

Insurance Contracts and Coverage

Health insurance contracts typically delineate the broad categories of services eligible for reimbursement, and specify exclude categories such as cosmetic surgery or unproven therapies. Yet insurers have generally not established detailed rules for determining the adequacy of evidence (Garber, 2001).

In practice, contractual language varies enormously, and definitions tend to be vague (e.g., "reasonable and necessary") and unpredictable (Garber, 2001). Contracts may call for coverage of "effective" therapies, for example, but there are few precise ways to define the boundaries of coverage, no unambiguous way to define "effective," and poor evidence and incomplete data in any case (Eddy, 2001). Eddy (2001) has written, "in general, existing contractual language is so flabby that it is almost worthless for creating accurate expectations, making decisions, avoiding disagreements, or settling disputes."

Over the years, a great deal of scrutiny has focused on conceptualizing and defining "medical necessity" (e.g., Daniels and Sabin, 1994; Rosenbaum et al., 1999; Singer and Bergthold, 2000; Studdert and Gresenz, 2002). However, the discussions have focused on *clinical* rather than cost-effectiveness issues.[3]

In recent years, health insurers have moved towards policies of "evidence-based coverage." In a broad sense, these policies promote value and comprise a kind of unstated cost-effectiveness rationale—in the sense that they call for explicit standards for determining effective care, thus avoiding payment for ineffective care (Garber, 2001). Eddy (2001) points out that the concept of cost-effectiveness is sometimes mentioned elliptically, buried in the notion of "appropriateness" or in language that speaks about the least expensive way to achieve an identical benefit. Others have found that if cost-effectiveness is addressed at all, it may be couched as "prudent use of plan resources" or the "most appropriate level of service" (Singer and Bergthold, 2001).

Few insurance contracts, if any, mention cost-effectiveness—or even cost for that matter—explicitly (Jacobson and Kanna, 2001). Some payers explicitly *exclude* its consideration—the State of California insurance regulations, for example, have required insurance to cover medically necessary goods and services and to provide health coverage to patients "unhindered by a plan's fiscal concerns" (Keith, 2000).

In theory, insurance contracts could state that insurers will cover services that are medically necessary *and cost-effective*. Why they do not is an interesting question that may in part be explained by their fear of litigation.

The Courts and Cost-Effectiveness

How the courts view cost-effectiveness analysis remains in many ways an unaddressed issue. To date there has been little litigation that directly raised or challenged the use of CEA (Jacobson and Rosenquist, 1988; Anderson et al., 1998; Jacobson and Kanna, 2001). Jacobson and Kanna (2001) note that inevitably such cases will arise and will turn on legal questions such as: Is evidence from CEAs admissible? What criteria will guide it? What is the weight of the evidence? What should patients be told? Should cost-effectiveness be treated as a standard of care or as another piece of evidence?

Some hint of the answers may come from how courts have handled other challenges to cost-containment tools used by managed-care organizations to limit medical treatments, such as utilization management, capitated funding arrangements, limitations on choice of providers and benefits, exclusive contractual arrangements, and other incentives, such as bonuses and salary withholds (Jacobson, 1999). So far, courts seem to have issued mixed rulings on challenges to managed-care plans' attempts to deny health benefits based on contractual limitations, sometimes ordering treatment, and sometimes not (Jacobson, 1999; Hall, 1999).

Though few insurers appear willing to go to court (Anderson et al., 1998), when they do, courts have sometimes overturned coverage decisions and sided with patients about whether expensive technologies should be covered, even if they are unproven (see Anderson, 1992; Ferguson et al,. 1993; Anderson et al., 1998; Jacobson, 1999; Mello and Brennan, 2001). Ferguson et al. (1993) point to several reasons for this, including ambiguities in the insurance contracts governing the "usual, customary, and reasonable" charges, the reluctance or inability of the courts to use the scientific literature, and the use of adversarial expert witnesses with conflicts of interest.

Anderson et al. (1993) notes the courts' traditional reluctance to accept medical technology assessment techniques.

Courts have tended to look to usual and customary practice in the industry or, in the absence of custom, to a "reasonableness" standard (Jacobson and Rosenquist, 1988). Jacobson and Kanna (2001) comment that the growing use of cost-containment measures could change what is considered customary. One might argue that a prevailing practice consti- tutes too *much* care, that "intensity does not necessarily equal *quality* of care." Plans could justify the use of CEAs to deny care to an individual patient by arguing that the provision of a service was not in the best interest of the population served, though the plaintiff could possibly argue that this was not based on sound methodology, or that it undervalued care, or was con- trary to stated plan criteria (Jacobson and Kanna, 2001).[4]

While contractual definitions such as "medical necessity" do not in- herently exclude cost-effectiveness considerations, plans may fear that patients would challenge its use if they were not informed about how it might influence clinical decisions (Jacobson and Kanna, 2001). Eddy (2001) notes the considerable room for misunderstanding and disagreement, given enormous variations in patients' conditions, histories, and behaviors, and the uncertainties surrounding treatment effects. He points out that there is no such thing as a community standard, that only retrospectively are consequences known, and that juries don't appreciate uncertainty prospectively.

Moreover, reluctance to use CEA may be attributable to fears about what *juries* might do. Concerns about jury reactions are borne out in inter- views with managed-care officials (Garber et al., 2000). In one survey of health plan officials, most respondents said they would approve equally effective but costlier treatments for fear of litigation or backlash (Singer, 1999). Plans for years reluctantly agreed to cover high-dose chemotherapy with autologous bone marrow transplant for breast cancer partly in response to the threat of litigation, despite its high cost and lack of evidence that it was effective (Mello and Brennan, 2001). Some physicians polled in an- other survey stated that because of malpractice concerns, they were hesi- tant to recommend anything but the most effective screening strategy regardless of cost (Ubel et al., 2003a).

Experience with the courts in non–health sectors may also make health plans hesitant about using CEA explicitly. Ford and General Motors were punished for using cost-benefit analysis to justify not installing safety- oriented designs, for example. Jacobson and Kanna (2001) point to the prob- lem of "smoking guns"—internal memos like those in the Ford and GM cases which could expose health plan officials and physicians to "withering cross-examination."

Hastie and Viscusi (1998) comment that when confronted *ex post facto* with real-life victims, jurors overestimate the *ex ante* risks (cited in Jacobson and Kanna, 2001). Eddy (2001) observes, "In some cases, an appeal to cost-effectiveness provides a successful defense; in others it kills a defendant's case. If there is a pattern at all, it appears to be that cost-effectiveness analysis is used when it can support the little guy against the big guy. To the extent that this is true, it is not very encouraging to health plans."

In the end, Americans' proclivity to sue may explain some of the reluctance by health plans to use cost-effectiveness analysis. Though legal scholars debate the issue (e.g., Jacobson and Rosenquist, 1988; Jacobson, 1999; Hall, 1999), there are also credible reasons to believe that managed-care plans could withstand legal challenges to the use of cost-effectiveness analysis, as they have withstood challenges to other cost-containment initiatives (Jacobson and Kanna, 2001). Courts have been disinclined to obstruct markets in organizing and delivering health care, and in general have been deferential to managed care (Eddy, 2001; Jacobson, 1999).[5] Similarly, nothing prevents the medical profession from factoring in resource constraints in defining which technology becomes customary, and courts have traditionally been reluctant to substitute their own judgment for the profession's (Jacobson and Rosenquist, 1988). Also, there are protections stemming from the Employee Retirement Income Security Act (ERISA) preemptions, which preclude patients from suing under state law for denial of care (Jacobson, 1999).

In addition, anticipation of court reaction does not seem to explain public payers' reluctance to use CEA, given that the courts have generally been more receptive to government application of CEA and CBA, and even encouraged it. Jacobson and Kanna (2001) argue that government agencies generally have wide latitude to use analytical tools such as cost-effectiveness analysis in their decision-making—that courts generally defer to regulatory agency experience, though decisions must be well reasoned, and not "arbitrary, capricious, an abuse of discretion, or otherwise not in accordance of the law." Even when courts find regulatory decisions arbitrary, they generally have remanded them to agencies for further consideration, leaving decision-making power to the agencies (though on occasion courts have questioned the methodology used) (Jacobson and Kanna, 2001).

The executive branch has on occasion been a strong proponent of CBA and CEA. President Reagan's Executive Order 12,291, revised in President Clinton's Executive Order 12,866, requires federal agencies to prepare a Regulatory Impact Analysis (RIA) for all major regulations, including the conduct of cost-benefit analyses to ensure that "benefits of the intended regulations justify their costs . . ." so that they are "to be designed in the most cost-effective manner" (*U.S. Federal Register*, 1981; *U.S. Federal Register*, 1993).[6] The Orders that authorize the Office of Management and Budget to oversee the process, state that federal agencies should consider both quantitative and qualitative measures (*U.S. Federal Register*, 1993). In its 2003 report to Congress on the costs and benefits of major health and safety regulations, OMB called for improving the technical quality of benefit-cost estimates and expanding the use of cost-effectiveness analysis as well as cost-benefit analysis in regulatory analyses (U.S. Office of Management and Budget, 2003).

All of these forces suggest that reluctance to use CEA in health and medicine may not reflect fears about courts and juries alone, but rather a larger fear about political or public relations backlash.

Political Barriers

Those who write about barriers to CEA often mention or imply a political component: that what private and public health officials and politicians fear above all is negative publicity, which may erode market share or jeopardize an election. At its roots, resistance to CEA may be grounded, not in methodological or institutional barriers, but in Americans' deep-seated distaste for limits and of the corporate or government officers who impose them. This well of public opinion may explain, as much as anything, the peculiar arc of American health policy—the mistrust of centralized technology assessment activities (Blumenthal, 1983; Deyo et al., 1997), the backlash against managed care (Blendon et al., 1998), and ultimately, resistance to the explicit use of CEA.

Survey data suggest that compared to their counterparts in Europe or Canada, Americans are more concerned about access to the most advanced medical technologies (Kim et al., 2001). Other countries' experiences with CEA confirm that the United States' failure to use CEA is driven more by its own cultural, political, and institutional conditions than by the technique's inherent methodological shortcomings.

This tendency was on display in the Pharmaceutical Research and Manufacturers of America (PhRMA's) reaction against proposed legislation in 2003 to authorize funding for NIH and the Agency for Health Care Research and Quality (AHRQ) to conduct additional CEAs. The argument was not against CEA per se, but against the government's use of the technique. "Cost-effectiveness analysis in the private sector can provide useful information," admitted PhRMA. "When employed by centralized decision-makers, however, it often becomes just another term for health care rationing" (cited in Pear, 2003). The letter went on to criticize "one size-fits-all-medicine" as bad for patients because it put the government in the position of directing medical decisions. Tellingly, the newly enacted Medicare drug legislation proposes new funds for "comparative effectiveness" not cost-effectiveness research by AHRQ, and explicitly forbids CMS to use the information to withhold coverage of new drugs (Medicare Prescription Drug, Improvement, and Modernization Act, 2003).

Embracing technological advances and rejecting limits remains a powerful tendency in American culture. There is a general dislike for limits. The application of CEA by public policy makers is framed by opponents as an initiative that would restrict freedom, impede access, and suppress innovation.

Eddy (1992a) has argued that people react to the overt nature of the CEA exercise itself, that it forces us to think at a conscious level about things we would much rather leave at a subconscious, private level. Rennie (2001) observes that the man in the street is highly skeptical of the value of tools such as cost-effectiveness analysis: "Their unpopularity is scarcely surprising, if only because when beliefs conflict with evidence, beliefs tend to win."

An ambitious effort in California to better define the role of cost-effectiveness as a criterion in treatment and coverage decisions, and to work "collaboratively, openly, inclusively, and realistically" toward solutions, underscored these points (Sacramento HealthCare, 2001). Consumers were generally not willing to accept cost-effectiveness as a reason for denying treatment for an individual patient. The consumers surveyed tended to believe that health plans could not fairly judge cost-effectiveness because plan managers cared more about cost than about effectiveness. Use of CEA reinforced the notion that decisions were made by bean-counters, not doctors. Moreover, consumers viewed private health-care coverage as an entitlement to an open set of benefits rather than a societal resource shared by many. Even their awareness of health costs did not translate into a willingness to conserve health-care resources they felt were owed to them.

A similar strain runs through American medicine, fueling a feeling that the commonly cited $50,000 per QALY[7] threshold for judging acceptable cost-effectiveness is too low (Ubel, Hirth, et al., 2003). A recent article in the *New England Journal of Medicine* concluded that the addition of clopidogrel for the secondary prevention of heart disease either alone or in combination with aspirin had an incremental cost of more than \$130,000/QALY gained at the current price of a 75-mg tablet of clopidogrel (\$3.22)—a cost described by the authors as "unattractive" (Gaspoz et al., 2002). Wood (2002) observed in an accompanying commentary that "the cost of the additional therapeutic benefits of clopidogrel is certainly high; however, to accept uncritically that it is 'unattractive' seems to me potentially dangerous." He went on to argue that society needs a continuing commitment to search for improved therapeutic strategies, and that to abandon the search for improved therapies would be an "enormous disservice to our patients." He concludes that with the overuse of CEA, "we are destined to be trapped at our current level of therapeutic efficacy forever, a very unattractive prospect."

In 1993, President Clinton's health reform team included an internal ethics task force that urged leadership to address rationing straightforwardly but they were instructed that the term "rationing" could not be used in any documents or memos (Daniels and Sabin, 2002). Interviews with managed-care executives reveal a grave fear that someone might accuse them of rationing. No one wants to be the first on the block to do it. Moreover, medical directors do not believe that they have the legitimacy to ration care in explicit ways because rationing represents a societal decision that private organizations cannot make (Daniels and Sabin, 2002).

Objections to CEA may be particularly acute in the United States given the country's for-profit health-care system. Consumers and providers may believe that these economically driven, sometimes publicly traded organizations are not motivated or inspired by a desire to maximize the value of health-care services to members of their plans. Furthermore, they may believe that the overall health system reflects an unwise and inefficient use of resources and are not motivated to forego potential beneficial care simply because of cost. People have demonized managed-care plans because they tried to limit patients' choice of provider and treatment based on economic considerations; they may view CEA as a formal, explicit methodology to achieve the same end (Neumann, 2004b).

Is CEA Fair?

An ethical critique

A related critique comes from medical ethicists and others who question CEA on the basis of equity and distributive justice, and who raise fundamental moral objections to conducting the exercise itself.

Cost-effectiveness as a guide to resource allocation, from society's perspective, is utilitarian. Benefits are maximized under given resource constraints for the population at large, with life years or QALYs as the agreed-upon measure of social benefit (Weinstein, 2001). Yet life years or QALYs may fail to capture public preferences for spending limited resources. Generally, this may reflect the fact that health is not the sole consideration in individual utility. The consumption of other goods and services also contributes to well-being (Gold et al., 1996, p. 31). Even taking into account health-care expenditures alone, people may not wish to maximize total returns in terms of QALYs. Instead, they may want to achieve other goals in setting priorities.[8]

For example, they may prefer interventions that help a few people gain a lot of health by giving priority to people most in need, to people suffering, or to certain vulnerable populations, such as children (Hadorn, 1991; Eddy 1992a; Nord, 1999; Ubel, 2000; Daniels and Sabin, 2002). The Oregon Medicaid program's decision in the 1980s to halt funding of transplants in order to redirect health resources to better uses was estimated to affect 34 unidentifiable lives in favor of providing basic health care to 1500 residents without health insurance. However, as Ubel (2000) notes, the fate of those 34 individuals weighs heavily upon us.

While intended as an empirical, transparent methodology relying on solid evidence, cost-effectiveness analysis is not value-neutral (Daniels and Sabin, 2000). It carries with it morally controversial and, to some, unacceptable assumptions. Chief among them is the assumption that a QALY is worth just as much, regardless of who benefits, which seems to violate a strong instinct to give priority to the sickest among us. Nord (1999) has argued that while there is increasing recognition that the assumption of distributive neutrality is not quite true, there is little awareness that it could be very wrong.

When should the aggregation of modest benefits to large numbers of people outweigh more substantial benefits to fewer people (Daniels, 1994)? Some distributions may be considered fairer than others (Nord, 1999). Cost-effectiveness analysts typically assign decrements in utility for minor ailments and disabilities. But as Kamm (1994) notes, will any number of sore throats cured equal saving a life? Criticizing a cost-utility analysis of sildenafil (Viagra) by Smith and Roberts (2000), McGregor (2003) remarks that one QALY gained by an otherwise healthy individual through the correction of erectile dysfunction would probably not be considered equivalent to a QALY gained by prolonging the life, by dialysis, of an individual about to die from renal failure.

QALYs also fail to capture the heterogeneity in preferences for health outcomes among subgroups. Researchers have long struggled with the question of how to reconcile diverse individual or subgroup preferences and values while applying CEA intended for population-wide decisions. Applying clinical standards to large groups rather than individuals seems at odds with good medical practice. "Accounting for individual variation is what medicine is all about," argued one policy expert not long ago in the *New England Journal of Medicine* (Rosenbaum et al., 1999). Applying population standards risks violating clinicians' advocacy duties, destroying the trust necessary for a good doctor–patient relationship (Ubel, 2000). Physicians' medical training emphasizes their ethical responsibility to patients for best available medical care, a responsibility that conflicts with their uncertain role as gatekeepers of limited resources for patients collectively (Weinstein, 2001). "When I am with a patient, I don't sit down with my calculator. As a physician, I want the best outcome," emphasized one physician in response to a question about rationing health care (Lagnado, 2003).

Some scholars have argued that as a society we actually do better by "muddling through carefully," rather than by explicitly allocating resources (Mechanic, 1997). Nord (1999) argues that "to rank projects in terms of cost per QALYs as often as not may tend to distort resource allocation decisions rather than to inform and aid them." Mechanic (1997) contends that explicit allocation, while seductive, is misleading and has the potential for mischief. He points to the difficulties involved in developing and changing explicit standards and the susceptibility of the process to political manipulations. He notes that medical care is a process of discovery and negotiation that requires flexibility and needs to account for patient differences in tastes and preferences, emotions and aspirations, not simply the application of technical means. He further argues that the value of implicit rationing lies in its capacity to respond to complexity, diversity, and changing information in a sensitive and timely way; that it offers the most meaningful path for thoughtful judgment consistent with the complexities of care.

Even CEA's proponents concede that the identification of subgroup preferences may be an important component to informing decision-making in resource allocation (Gold et al., pp. 102–3).[9] When and how to do it is much less clear. The *Panel* comments that a person with terminal illness may place a high value on living until a particular milestone reached (such as a child's wedding), but such idiosyncrasies are not captured when CEA is applied at the population level (Gold et al., 1996, p. 34). Williams (1997) has argued that resource-allocation decisions should discriminate against the elderly according to a "fair innings" basis; that is, on the notion that people are entitled to a "normal" lifetime of around 70 to 75 years, and that the people attaining more than this are living on borrowed time.

Finally, some object to the entire enterprise of CEA on the general philosophical grounds that it amounts to a mindless pursuit of efficiency or that it is wrong to attempt to quantify health benefits that are not easily quantified, that "numbers don't tell us everything" (Heinzerling and Ackerman, 2002). Application of CEA is seen as violating the special moral importance of health, or as breaching citizens' inherent rights to health care (Daniels and Sabin, 2002). Two leading critics have written that it transforms the discussion from one of rights and ethics into a complex, resource-intensive, and expert-driven process that produces a number, which obscures the debate about underlying values (Heinzerling and Ackerman, 2002). They add that the process of reducing life, health, and the natural world to monetary values is inherently flawed, that it turns public citizens into selfish consumers. Elsewhere, they argue that the process of discounting future costs and benefits can trivialize long-term risks (Heinzerling and Ackerman, 2002). Others note that CEA ignores social goals, such as the desire to protect people against financial risk, or spending in favor of the poor (Hutubessy et al., 2002; Murray et al., 2000).

Empirical evidence on how people want to allocate public resources

Empirical evidence suggests that QALYs may not account for people's actual preferences for rationing and priority-setting in health care.

Patients, and their physicians, seem to want equity and fairness in a general sense, rather than efficiency per se (Ubel et al., 1998a; Ubel et al., 1998b; Ubel, 2000; Perneger et al., 2002). While they would like to save as many lives as possible, they also want to give people hope and to ensure access to all, even if their prognosis is poor. They also want to avoid discrimination against people with chronic illness or disability even when treatments are not cost-effective (Ubel, 2000, pp. 76, 78–85). People tend to believe that equally ill persons should have the same right to treatment irrespective of whether the treatment effect is large or moderate. Nord (1999) argues that evidence shows people are not even health maximizers behind their veil of ignorance. He points to strong empirical evidence that the severity of patients' illness matters. The amount of benefit provided to those worse off seems to matter a great deal.

In one survey, subjects placed a value on treating severely ill people that was tenfold to one-hundred-thousand-fold greater than would have been predicted by utility responses (Ubel et al., 1996). Another survey of physicians reported that respondents generally thought that cost-effectiveness was an appropriate criterion when making treatment decisions for their patients, but were divided on whether they had a duty to offer all treatment options when "the chance of success was small and the cost was great" (Ginsberg et al., 2000). In other surveys of physicians, some respondents made moral arguments against basing clinical recommendations on cost-effectiveness (Ubel et al., 2003a).

Conclusion

CEA promises to inform decisions and enhance population health in an explicit, quantitative and systematic manner. Yet various factors have conspired to create resistance to its explicit use for priority-setting in the United States: a lack of understanding about the conceptual approach, a mistrust of methods, a mistrust of motives, and ethical, regulatory, and legal barriers.

Each of these explanations also has shortcomings. Lack of understanding or mistrust of methods and motives undoubtedly play a role. Still, why haven't policy makers in the United States funded or conducted their own CEAs or tailored them to their own needs as they have in other countries?

Legal and regulatory factors also fail as a full explanation. Nothing in the federal statutes explicitly bars Medicare from using CEA. Similarly, nothing prevents private health insurers from writing contracts that specify covered services as those that are deemed "medically necessary and cost-effective." Plans may fear lawsuits if they use cost-effectiveness openly. But there are also plausible reasons to believe that health plans could withstand these challenges, as they have withstood challenges to other cost-containment initiatives.

The best explanation is that, at its roots, resistance to CEA in the United States is grounded, not in methodological or legal barriers, but in Americans' penchant for medical innovation and our distaste for limits—and in our deep-rooted suspicion of governments or corporations that impose them.

These factors were on full display in American health care's one great experiment with explicit priority-setting using cost-effectiveness, which took place in Oregon over a number of years in the late 1980s and early 1990s. The manner in which CEA was used and finally abandoned in the Oregon Medicaid plan provides a unique window through which to view the debate. I turn to its lessons in the next chapter.

6

Lessons from Oregon

. . . .

We had a rational policy. Now it was a tough policy, and there were tough decisions that were made and I'm not saying people didn't get hurt, but at least we were honest about it.

—John Kitzhaber, former Oregon state representative
and governor, 2003

The Oregon Experiment

Oregon's experiment with cost-effectiveness was part of a grander proposal to overhaul the state's health insurance system, which included several features: requiring employers to provide health insurance to all permanent employees, funding a high-risk pool for individuals with preexisting conditions, and expanding the state's Medicaid program to cover additional state residents.

The Medicaid expansion was to be paid for by enrolling new Medicaid recipients in managed care and by restricting the standard benefit package provided. The state planned to limit benefits by: (1) developing a prioritized list of paired medical conditions and treatments that ranked the value of services from most important to least important, according to information on their costs and effects, and (2) covering only the services that fell above a line established by the state's budgetary resources.

The Oregon plan quickly became the subject of intense debate. Proponents held that the plan would enable the state to provide health insurance to many more low-income residents, and that it was a more rational way of apportioning limited resources. In addition to praising the boldness of the idea, advocates lauded the public and participatory nature of the process, a "classic exercise of American democracy in the sunlight" (Daniels, 1991; Fox and Leichter, 1991; Leichter, 1999). It involved elected officials, community leaders, and health professionals who came together to define an adequate minimum standard of health care, in a manner that was seen as politically accountable, that reflected community values, and that was subject to the vote of the legislature (Fox and Leichter, 1991). Ultimately, eleven public hearings were held around the state. Advocates argued that even if it had problems, the plan represented a useful starting point for an intelligent debate (Eddy, 1991). John Kitzhaber, the physician and state senator (and later governor) who ushered the plan through the Oregon legislature, said "Our detractors consist mainly of uninformed members of threatened interest groups who delight in comparing the Oregon plan to a perfect world" (cited in Fox and Leichter, 1991).

In contrast, critics—including U.S. Senator Albert Gore, U.S. Representative Henry Waxman, and groups ranging from the Children's Defense fund and the American Academy of Pediatrics to the National Association of Community Health Centers, U.S. Catholic Conference, and the National Association of Children's Hospitals (Brown, 1991)—attacked the plan for unfairly singling out the state's poorest citizens for the rationing scheme.[1] Medicaid recipients would be denied medically necessary services that fell "below the line." The plan was criticized for discriminating on the basis of class, age, race, and sex (because Medicaid recipients are disproportionately poor, young, nonwhite, and female). One pair of critics called it politically convenient and ethically execrable (Himmelstein and Woolhandler, 1998). Some argued that the process was neither open nor fair, because the poor were not represented (Daniels, 1991; Jacobs et al., 1999). The Children's Defense Fund argued that the process amounted to 1000 healthy upper-middle-class people making decisions for poor children on what services to take away (Brown, 1991).

The Role of Cost-Effectiveness

The actual role of cost-effectiveness analysis was often lost in the rhetoric. Some criticized the process either generally as "garbage in/garbage out," or specifically for its heavy emphasis on costs (Brown, 1991). In an implicit swipe at the cost-effectiveness methodology, Senator Gore said the plan represented "playing God by playing with spreadsheets." Bruce Vladeck, who would later head HCFA, called it a "misbegotten mishmash of second-rate policy analysis and cynical budgetary politics" (cited in Brown, 1991). An official at the Children's Defense Fund complained that "the methodological basis for this is insane" (cited in Bodenheim, 1997).

In a few cases, critics attacked the methodology explicitly. Notably, David Hadorn (1991) argued in the *Journal of the American Medical Association* (JAMA) that cost-effectiveness analysis was inherently flawed, and that it was incapable of capturing the value people place on lifesaving technologies and on rescuing individual, identifiable lives.

Proponents of the plan countered that the cost-effectiveness methodology was crude but refinable. They pointed to other methodologies used in health policy—diagnosis-related groups (DRGs) and the resource-based relative value scale (RBRVS)—as examples of technically complex but workable policy measures (Eddy, 1991; Brown, 1991).

In the end, though, formal CEA itself played little role in the actual plan. It proved so controversial and difficult to implement that it was abandoned early on in the process even as the priority list was salvaged. Oregon's first ranked list, released in May 1990 using a formula to estimate the cost-effectiveness of treatments, was widely criticized within the state because of counterintuitive rankings (e.g., tooth-capping ranked above surgery for ectopic pregnancy, and splints for temporomandibular joints ranked higher than appendectomies). The list was never submitted to the Health Care Financing Administration for approval (Brown, 1991; Eddy, 1991; Tengs et al., 1996).[2]

A second list, which modified the first one in numerous ways, such as rearranging the rankings on the basis of expert judgment rather than explicit appeals to cost and benefit information, was subsequently submitted to HCFA. This list also amended the ranking approach, by assigning treatment/condition pairs to 17 categories (e.g., "treatments that prevented death with full recovery," "maternity care," "treatments that caused minimal or no improvement in quality of life") according to values, such as "essential to basic health care," "value to an individual," and "value to society" (Tengs et al., 1996). This version was rejected in 1992 by the federal agency on the grounds that it violated the Americans with Disabilities Act (ADA). The rejection was based on two factors: (1) that quality-of-life measures were based on the preferences of healthy individuals, rather than those with disabilities; and (2) that the disabled could be discriminated against under the plan, because treatments which restored such individuals to their "normal" disabled state could be undervalued relative to those who returned to a "healthy" state.

Ultimately, a third, further amended list, which addressed the ADA concerns, was approved by HCFA in 1993 (after additional modifications to the list that gave more weight to the judgments of Commissioners in assigning rankings), and the plan was enacted in 1994.[3]

The Plan's Impact

Effects on access

Some have called the Oregon plan, which eventually took effect in 1994, a success because the state ultimately succeeded in expanding its Medicaid program (Bodenheim, 1997). Moreover, it has been argued that despite the controversy it provoked and ongoing budgetary struggles that followed, the plan has proved politically durable and even popular, and represented an important, symbolic departure from "do-everything-possible medicine" (Bodenheim, 1997; Jacobs et al., 1999; Leichter, 1999). It shifted the focus of health policy debates from considerations about which *populations* to cover to which *benefits* (Leichter, 1999). It has been argued that few serious complaints about its prioritized list emerged, and to the extent that problems arose, they were similar to problems in states around the country (Bodenheim, 1997).

The Oregon Health Plan (OHP) did add over 100,000 residents a year to its Medicaid rolls (a 25% increase), enrolling most in managed-care plans. The number of uninsured Oregonians declined during the first few years of program, at time when the uninsured numbers rose in the rest of country (Bodenheim, 1997; Haber et al., 2000).[4] The availability of health insurance, and possibly the greater use of managed-care plans, seem to have increased the utilization of health-care services and reduced unmet need for care among enrollees; for example, enrollees were likelier to have a usual source of care and higher rates of Pap test screening compared to similar populations not enrolled (Mitchell et al., 2002a).

Yet Oregon's efforts to prioritize services came at a high price, monetarily and politically. Eligibility and benefit expansions more than offset any restricted access that might have accompanied mandatory managed-care and the priority list. The state offered a generous benefit package, with expanded coverage for dental care and drugs and full integration of mental health and chemical dependency services into the basic package, along with integration of the elderly and disabled below the poverty line (Bodenheim, 1997; Ham, 1998; Leichter, 1999). Overall, Medicaid expenditures rose 39% in Oregon in the three years following enactment, as opposed to 30% nationally (Bodenheim, 1997). The plan was paid for from general revenues and a tobacco tax, as well as some savings through managed care (Jacobs et al., 1999).

As far as the priority list itself was concerned, one evaluation found no evidence that "rationing" under the list substantially reduced access to needed services (Mitchell et al., 2002a). Indeed, researchers have found higher use of certain services, such as mammograms, after the plan was enacted, as well as greater use of dental care and prescription drugs, compared to other low-income insured populations (Leichter, 1999; Mitchell et al., 2002a; Mitchell et al., 2000b). While studies did uncover an unmet need for prescription drugs, researchers attributed it more to the fact that a specific drug was simply not in a plan's formulary than to below-the-line conditions being denied (Mitchell et al., 2002a).

One evaluation found that, in general, OHP enrollees were as satisfied with their care as other low-income, private insurance recipients in Oregon (Mitchell et al., 2002a). Only 10% stated that they did not receive care because the doctor said the service was "below the line," including TMJ splints and treatment of back problems, such as physical therapy and chiropractic care (Mitchell et al., 2002a). Researchers also found that the priority list affected only 2% of children, most of whom succeeded in receiving care anyway (Mitchell et al., 2002b). Very few OHP recipients have appealed decisions for denial of services, which they may do under the plan (Leichter, 1999), and even beneficiaries who were denied a service that they thought they needed reported high levels of satisfaction with OHP (Mitchell and Bentley, 2000).

In the end, few services seem to have actually been rationed, as the initial line was set quite low to begin with (Bodenheim, 1997). According to one estimate, the list only saved 2% of total costs over five years (Jacobs et al., 1999). Bodenheim (1997) points out that certain very expensive therapies received high (i.e., favorable) rankings—such as renal transplantation for end-stage renal disease (ESRD), and liver transplantation for biliary atresia and other life-threatening hepatic disorders—and that in some cases coverage was more generous before the OHP. Moreover, many services that might have seemed targets were ranked favorably. Examples include contraception, which ranked at line 51 out of roughly 700 treatment/condition pairs; treatment of low-birth-weight newborns (under 2500g) at line 67; and preventive services for children at line 143 (Bodenheim, 1997). The main exclusions were for clinically marginal or ineffective therapies or for self-limiting conditions (Ham, 1998; Leichter, 1999).

Some evidence also indicates that "below-the-line" services continue to be provided as physicians "game" the system (M. Gold et al., 1996; Bodenheimer, 1997; Jacobs et al., 1999; Kilborn, 1999; Leichter, 1999; Mitchell and Bentley, 2000). Doctors have found several ways around the rationing scheme; for example, by changing the diagnosis and moving a condition from below to above the line (Kilborn, 1999), or by coding co-morbid conditions that would permit funding (Leichter, 1999). Sometimes they have simply provided the below-the-line treatment at the time of the diagnostic visit (Bodenheim, 1997). In a survey of 1400 Medicaid beneficiaries in Oregon, one-third reported needing a service that Medicaid would not cover, but in only 38% of these cases was the reason reported to be that the service was below the line (Mitchell and Bentley, 2000). About half of the individuals denied services reported receiving the service anyway, though often by paying for it themselves (Mitchell and Bentley, 2000).

Moreover, amid repeated spending increases and budget shortfalls, state policy makers have been more inclined to limit the number of *individuals* covered than to move the priority line to further restrict *services* (Kilborn, 1999).[5] State Medicaid officials have argued that such eligibility changes were necessary because federal Medicare officials would never approve a waiver that restricted services to the degree required to rebalance the plan (Leichter, 1999; Kilborn, 1999; Goldsmith, 2003).[6]

Moreover, only a fraction (as low as 13%) of Oregon's Medicaid fee-for-service patients have been subject to scrutiny about the actual threshold. Other populations have shifted to health plans that provide more flexibility to physicians for individual decisions (Bodenheim, 1997; Ham, 1998). One study found that OHP beneficiaries in managed-care plans were significantly more likely than those in fee for service to receive an uncovered service: 32% vs. 25% (Mitchell and Bentley, 2000). While the state does take away a proportion of payment it says goes for below-the-line treatments, plans often cover these services anyway–for example, they cover treatments for minor and inexpensive unfunded conditions, such as skin problems (Leichter, 1999), or even high-dose chemotherapy and BMT for a 9-year-old with medulloblastoma, a $75,000 treatment of unproven efficacy below the line (Bodenheim, 1997).

Take-Home Lessons for Cost-Effectiveness Analysis

Many in the health policy community greeted the idea of the Oregon plan, and its incorporation of cost-effectiveness analysis, with great fanfare and expectations. This would be the model for future efforts, one that incorporated fairness, transparency, and most of all, an explicit recognition of society's limits.

No other state ever emulated the model, however. Nor, for that matter, have other Western democracies, all of which manage to cover their populations without Oregon's "apocalyptic debate on rationing" (Brown, 1991).[7]

Instead, they have dealt with the same problems without the "combustible" priority list, in part by eliminating certain benefits, but mostly by redefining eligibility, reducing reimbursement to providers, and rapidly expanding managed-care options (Fox and Leichter, 1991; Bodenheimer, 1997; Gold, 1997). As for cost-effectiveness analysis, even Oregon discarded it early in its process.

Why then did CEA fail in Oregon?

Technical problems

Some have pointed to problems with the methodology (Eddy 1991; Ubel, 2000). Even as Oregon dismantled the cost-effectiveness methodological basis of the plan, some proponents continued to applaud the effort and insist that the failure was technical rather than conceptual in nature, that the task was "just too big for the available data and methods" (Eddy, 1992c), and that Oregon did not fail because people were opposed to rationing as such (Ubel, 2000, p. 47).

Among the technical problems noted by the Oregon Commission itself were: that condition and treatment pairs were defined too broadly, that duration of benefits of treatment was inaccurately estimated, and that cost data were incomplete or inaccurate (Eddy, 1991). Eddy (1992d) faulted the crudeness of the methodology: "attempting it forces analysts to aggregate treatments and indications to such a high degree and to apply such crude measures of benefits and costs that errors are inevitable, results become suspect, and process is difficult to defend."

Another argument was that the list didn't reflect genuine cost-effectiveness analysis at all, that there was almost no relationship between the 1990 list and cost-effectiveness estimates from the economic literature, and only a modest positive relationship between the 1991–1993 lists and published cost-effectiveness estimates (Tengs et al., 1996). Indeed, a study found that there was little relationship between the 1991–1993 lists and Oregon's own cost-effectiveness data (Tengs et al., 1996). The 1993 list was ranked primarily by improvement in five-year survival as well as adjustments made by human judgment, not cost-effectiveness data.

A possible explanation points to problems with the method for estimating preference weights in calculating quality-adjusted life years gained, because it relied on a rating-scale methodology, rather than "choice" methods, such as time tradeoff or standard gamble techniques, which involve asking respondents to value health states by explicitly considering how much they would be willing to sacrifice to avoid being in a particular state with impaired health (Gold et al., 1996). Others have argued that the methods used focused attention on health outcomes rather than the attributes of the services that may affect the outcome, or that they failed to capture the need to incorporate "vicarious" utilities—the desirability of outcomes to people other than the patient—e.g., how much utility they as bystanders would receive for saving an identifiable person from death from cancer (Ubel, 2000).

Most generally, some experts have argued, the plan failed to capture public rationing preferences in ways useful for setting health-care priorities. As Ubel (1996) has noted, people's answers to utility elicitation questions cannot be easily translated into social policy. Questions asked from the point of view of the individual, not society, may fail to capture how individuals felt about a collection of symptoms, and may fail to reflect how the public wishes to allocate different types of treatments across individuals (Ubel, 2000).

Moreover, Oregon-style priority-setting approaches open themselves up to charges of discrimination (Hadorn, 1992). The Oregon telephone survey to elicit preference weights to be used in QALY estimates did not make any special effort to include disabled people. The argument is that medical outcomes expected in disabled individuals and the values they place on those outcomes may be different from the general public's (Hadorn, 1992). Therefore, treatment that restores someone to a disabled state (e.g., selective treatment of very low birth weight infants) might not be valued fairly under the plan (Hadorn, 1992).

Political problems

The Panel on Cost-Effectiveness commented that Oregon's "bold effort" fell victim to political factors as well as methodological ones (Gold et al., p. vii). The argument that has gained currency in some quarters was that the State of Oregon, and the country at large, simply wasn't ready for the innovative approach; that the plan was ahead of its time. David Eddy (1992c) remarked, "I don't believe that the methodology . . . is sufficiently well developed to try to determine the effectiveness and cost of all the important medical treatments, for all their possible indications. Although in theory that might be possible, and although in principle it is the right thing to do, it is not a practical possibility yet." Others have commented that, as a country, we haven't sorted out our feelings about rationing, but that this doesn't necessarily mean any attempt will fail (Ubel, 2000, p. 10).

But a better case can be made that the failure of explicit priority-setting using cost-effectiveness analysis reveals a more fundamental and far-reaching political breakdown. In the twelve years since the original list, no state ever attempted to address the technical problems. No state has tried, in any formal or systematic way, to sort out its own feelings about rationing in Oregon-style fashion. No one has ever seriously proposed an Oregon plan for Medicare, "the most inviting and logical target" (Brown, 1991). If they have considered it at all, policy makers and legislators have probably shuddered at the thought of going through the process, with its promise of political turmoil and haggling over where to draw the line, not to mention higher spending, when there are other ways to achieve the same goals. At least for the current generation, and perhaps for the next several, the Oregon plan's main political legacy may be its enduring lessons about how *not* to make policy. A decade after its inception, it already seems like the high-water mark of the rationalists who would use cost-effectiveness analysis mechanistically to allocate resources in health care.

While Oregon zigged, the rest of the country zagged, adopting utilization controls and other management techniques. Vladeck (2000) has commented that a decade later, Oregon's whole approach from the early 1990s seems rather quaint. In his view, the principle that one can generate funds to cover people by reducing volume of services came true, but through managed care. Ironically, affluent Oregonians themselves became subject to more arbitrary and stringent limitations on access through the policies of HMOs, rather than Oregon's explicit rationing scheme.

In the end, even Oregon didn't come close to implementing cost-effectiveness analysis. The technocratic vision failed (Jacobs et al., 1999). Adjustments to the list were ultimately made, not based on CEA, but "by hand," on the basis of judgments by Oregon's Health Services Commission, and only then after a major overhaul to satisfy federal requirements and opposition to rankings. If anything, Oregon forced a discussion about medical necessity rather than cost-effectiveness (Vladeck, 2000). It opened a window on American values and the country's deeply felt unease toward confronting limits. Even in Oregon, the worst fears and tough choices never materialized (Jacobs et al., 1999).

Instead of offering a crucible for providing lessons about CEA, Oregon became a vessel into which critics could pour their grievances about the American health care system in general. As Brown (1991) has noted, the Oregon plan was "less instructive to policymakers than to sociologists seeking curious sub-national variations on American folkways," that it was "an exotic object of fascination addressed in luncheon symposiums and after-dinner speeches. . . ." As others have observed, rather than providing a genuine model, Oregon became a vehicle for ethicists, policy makers, legislators, activists, and health professionals of all ideologies to criticize their health-care system (Jacobs et al., 1999, Leichter, 1999).

Some scholars have even argued that for Oregon, the plan was about the process itself, a case study in participatory democracy, aiming to show that the state was capable of open-door policies and innovative social policy (Fox and Leichter, 1991). Both the Bush I and Clinton Administrations extolled the virtues of states as laboratories, especially with state-administered Medicaid programs, and favored the idea of Oregon's experimenting, if not the experiment itself. Federal policy makers could do so with little electoral consequence (Brown, 1991). Ham (1998) remarks that outsiders also loved the innovation for its own sake: Oregon won the Innovations in American Government prize by the Ford Foundation in 1996, for example.

Oregon also became more a forum for debate about inefficiencies in the health-care system and its lack of universal coverage, than about cost-effectiveness analysis as such. Its chief proponent, John Kitzhaber, wanted in particular to expose and address existing shortfalls in the health-care system.

To an extent the plan succeeded in that goal. Though the employer mandate was never enacted,[8] the state did establish insurance pools for small business and high-risk groups. Leichter (1999) points out that the plan shifted the political debate to let legislatures see what services they were covering, that it provided a "benefits perspective" on health care, and that the plan was a useful political tool as a vehicle for calculating the amount the state would invest in Medicaid each year.

It has been argued that the political calculation over rationing in Oregon worked, that in fact the rhetoric and the *process* of rationing—as distinct from its actual programmatic application—were crucial in mobilizing support for the Oregon Health Plan (OHP) and in pressuring the legislature to expand access without significantly reducing services; that in fact it made actual rationing less, not more, likely (Jacobs et al. 1999). Jacobs et al. (1999) argue that the discussion about rationing kept stakeholders directly engaged, and that the ultimate innovation in Oregon was more political than technical in nature. Others have made the case that the Oregon plan, like all innovations in public policy, succeeded when incremental in nature (Leicter, 1999).

But these arguments seem too clever. Oregon's proponents believed in the methods. Indeed, the methods provided the plan's centerpiece, and to its advocates gave it its legitimacy.

While it is true that the rationing plan mobilized support and pressured the legislature, it came at a high price. And the idea was never transportable across state lines (Jacobs et al., 1999). In the end, Oregon was emblematic above all about the limits of explicit rationing. It was an important policy experiment, but only in the way that public policy, like science, advances through trial and error and experimentation. The process requires its blind alleys and Oregon provided an important one at least for late 20th century America.

More than anything, Oregon exposed the limits of publicly applying explicit rationing policies in the United States today. It revealed in part the risks of broad citizen participation—which some called a "politically and legally flawed strategy to gain widespread acceptance for innovative reform" (Fox and Leichter, 1993). As Brown (1991) has remarked, the "voice of the people is too vague to speak clearly to concrete coverage decisions."

More important, it revealed the challenges of overly prescriptive health policy. The specificity of the list can become a political albatross (Fox, Leichter, 1993). Vladeck (2000) commented that "the nation's health policy community, dominated by practitioners of quantitative disciplines particularly ill-suited to understanding the social roles of professionalism, and the psychosocial dimensions of physician–patient relations, may be institutionally incapable of providing much help to policy makers."

Ironically, drawing up a list served inevitably to define and *inflate* the basic health-care package, rather than functioning as a strict rationing instrument (Ham, 1998; Jacobs et al., 1999). The process in Oregon produced a more generous package of benefits than what Medicaid or the private sector had offered before, as the legislature added or expanded benefits for mental health or HIV coverage, for example (Jacobs et al., 1999). It also served to define a floor of coverage for everyone in the state (Fox, Leichter, 1993).

The plan exposed the limits of CEA as a practical, acceptable means of formulaic priority-setting for a generation of health policy makers and politicians. The use of CEA not only attracted criticism, it also added to state health costs. Ultimately, it did not prove a feasible way to make policy.

Hadorn (1991) cites an early argument in favor of CEA, which held that while the equitable distribution of benefits and costs among individuals was a concern, it was likely to even itself out over a large number of programs so that, with some exceptions, they might reasonably be ignored (Weinstein and Stason, 1977). Oregon demonstrated that distributional issues cannot reasonably be ignored. As Hadorn (1991) noted, the most fundamental lesson to be learned from the Oregon experience was that use of cost-effectiveness analysis was unlikely to produce a socially or politically acceptable definition of necessary care. Most notably, this finding was at odds with opinions expressed by most health economists and by most health scholars.

As of 2003, Oregon policy makers continued to refine their system.[9] But its priority-setting scheme remains an exception. And it still does not incorporate cost-effectiveness analysis formally. Moreover, the plan again is confronting serious budgetary challenges, attributable in part to larger economic conditions, but also to rising health-care costs. As the legislature again seeks to come up with the money, it seems loath to move the prioritization line and has begun charging some people higher monthly premiums and new co-payments.

Perhaps most important of all, the Oregon Medicaid program has recently implemented an evidence-based process to consider drugs for its preferred drug list. The process involves detailed public reviews of various therapeutic classes. After completing the clinical reviews, the Medicaid agency considers the prices of drugs deemed clinically equivalent or for which there is a lack of evidence to indicate one drug's effectiveness over another (Kaiser Commission on Medicaid and the Uninsured, 2004). As of early 2004, eight other states are collaborating with Oregon to share the costs and use the results of the reviews. The role of cost considerations remains controversial. But the model is instructive both because it does not appeal to rigid cost-effectiveness rankings, and because it reveals what may emerge as an acceptable use of economic information, as discussed at greater length in chapters 7 and 10.

Conclusion

CEA's proponents have always assumed that rising spending and the public's appetite for medical technology will eventually force our society to recognize limits more directly, and that inevitably, we will use formal CEA as the best solution to our dilemma.

Yet in the face of rising health-care spending, the resistance to acknowledging limits—and using CEA—has proven remarkably durable. There is no groundswell of support among policy makers or politicians for using the approach. Instead, the idea of explicit rationing has been shoved far under the table. In retrospect, the application of CEA in Oregon cut in fundamental ways against the grain of American values. The Oregon plan attracted untoward attention from health policy makers, but not because it ever provided a realistic model for reform. In the end, no one attempted to adopt Oregon's plan to use CEA—not even Oregon. Rather than serving as a roadmap for health policy, Oregon functioned ultimately as a kind of national sounding board, a vehicle for expressing grievances with the American health-care system at large. It revealed more than anything the resistance to openly confronting limits.

Medicare today still does not use costs or cost-effectiveness explicitly as criteria in making coverage decisions. Robinson (2001) has observed that Medicare is popular as long as there are no visible restrictions on choices. He notes that governmental entities avoid politically volatile initiatives to balance limited resources. "No one even whispers that public resources are limited" (Robinson, 2001). Rather, in times of deficits, they cut payments to providers and reassure the voting public that there are no sacrifices.

In the private sector, health plans have opted to employ other management tools than CEA. Managed care's protagonists have lately been in full retreat, broadening physician panels, removing restrictions, and reverting to fee-for-service payments (Robinson, 2001). The most notable trend has been consumerism, fueled by widespread skepticism of governmental, corporate and professional dominance (Robinson, 2001).

But how to explain the fact that medical journals, including the most prestigious ones, routinely publish CEAs? How to reconcile "resistance" with the fact that many other countries have incorporated CEA explicitly into their technology assessment and reimbursement procedures? I turn to these questions in the next chapters.

7

Does Anyone in America Really Use CEA? Examples from the Field

. . . .

> *If an [implantable cardiac defibrillator] were a buck and a quarter, would*
> *we have gone through this entire process of reviewing the evidence at all?*
> *Maybe not. But because it's a bit more than a buck and a quarter we*
> *wanted to make sure the evidence was clear and that it was a benefit. We*
> *don't use cost to decide the evidence issue, but we do use cost to decide if*
> *this is important enough to address.*
>
> —Steve Phurrough, the acting director of the CMS Coverage
> and Analysis Group, 2003

Cost-Effectiveness in the Ether

The resistance to CEA highlighted in chapters 3 through 6 suggests that the technique has had little impact. CEA might be characterized as an elegant but forbidden tool, beautifully made but outlawed as too dangerous. Still, the possibility remains that CEA actually enjoys considerable influence, not as an explicit instrument for prioritizing health services, but as a subtler input into decision making.

The avalanche of CEAs in the medical literature lends weight to this argument. Between 1975 and 2000, researchers published many thousands of economic evaluations of health care[1] in peer-reviewed health and medical journals. By the late 1990s, almost 100 cost/life year or cost/QALY studies were being published each year. Most appeared in general medical and specialty journals and were written by investigators from the United States (Neumann et al., 2000; www.hsph.harvard.edu/cearegistry) (Fig. 7–1). The studies covered a bewildering array of intervention types and diseases and conditions.[2] By the dawn of the twenty-first century, cost-effectiveness analysts had carved out a distinctive place in mainstream academic American medicine, even as the studies' impacts remained elusive.

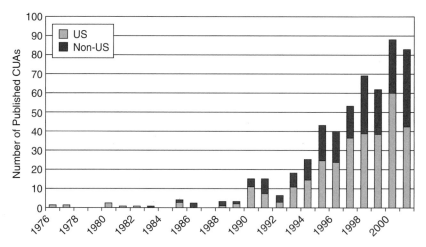

Figure 7–1.   Growth in published CUAs, 1976–2001. *Source*: CEA Registry, Harvard School of Public Health, 2003 (www.hsph.harvard.edu/cearegistry).

Why would analysts continue publishing studies if the information was being ignored in policy designs? Their motive may have been to influence the general tenor of the debate. A CEA may serve to influence opinion on a subject or simply add to the weight of information on an intervention (Gold et al., 1996, p. 58). CEAs may serve most usefully as a navigational tool rather than an explicit decision-making instrument (Powers and Eisenberg, 1998).

As the *Panel on Cost-Effectiveness* argues, the structured process of conducting CEAs—of evaluating the strength of evidence, stating assumptions, and working on implications—can be as helpful as the final estimates (Gold et al., p. 10). Over the years, CEA has helped challenge prevailing wisdom and has brought clarity to health policy debates, underscoring, for example, that prevention programs usually do not produce cost savings (Russell, 1986); that high-tech, cost-increasing interventions can sometimes provide very good value for money (Weinstein, 1999); and that an additional diagnostic test can be enormously expensive relative to the clinical benefits conferred (Neuhauser and Lewicki, 1975).

A prime example is screening tests. How frequently to screen, which tests to use, and which populations to cover are all questions that require physicians to think about costs and cost-effectiveness (Ubel, 2000, p. 26). Textbooks have long maintained that such tests should be inexpensive and should detect common and curable disease: in other words, they should be cost-effective (Eddy, 1991; Ubel, 2000, p. 142). Formal CEAs in the late

1980s and early 1990s to quantify the costs and benefits associated with specific screening strategies helped shape the medical community's recognition that screening for cancer every, say, two years was a rational policy given resource constraints, even if one could detect more cancers with more frequent screening (Eddy, 1989; 1990a, 1990b).

In a broad way much of health policy constitutes a search for cost-effective care. Over the years, cost-effectiveness analyses have become an integral part of the messy jumble of evidence that seeps into clinical guidelines and diffuses into broader definitions of accepted medical practice. As far back as 1980, a study found that more than 65 pieces of proposed federal legislation related to health included words such as "cost-effectiveness" and "cost-effective medical care" (cited in Warner and Luce, 1982). A more recent study showed good concordance between rankings of the appropriateness of medical technology in certain applications (e.g., coronary angiography after myocardial infarction) and the cost-effectiveness ratios for these indications (Kuntz et al., 1999)

Cholesterol screening is another good example. Statin drugs used to lower an individual's cholesterol have been found to be relatively cost-effective as secondary prevention in persons with existing heart disease, but considerably less cost-effective as primary prevention (Goldman et al., 1991). While formal recommendations published by the NIH's National Cholesterol Education Program (NCEP) didn't follow the CEAs strictly, the economic analyses were cited in the guidelines (NCEP, 1994). And while health plans and practicing physicians may not admit to using CEA to exclude certain population segments from statin treatment (or even understand that at some level they do incorporate this information), the analyses probably play a role in this practice (Gold et al., 1996, pp. 15–18, 58).

The reach of CEA may similarly extend into most areas of health policy making. While decision makers have shunned explicit application of the technique, this hasn't thwarted CEA's influence so much as recast the way it is exerted and disseminated.

Pharmaceutical companies, for example, have actively used pharmaco-economic models as inputs into pricing strategies and key development and marketing decisions. Drug company researchers have used the information to predict the price that authorities should be willing to pay for a new drug product, based on its potential costs and benefits. For a particular price that plan managers know has to be achieved for commercial viability, preliminary analysis may show what level of efficacy or what sales profile is required for a product to be cost-effective at that price (Clemens, Garrison et al., 1993).

If anything, recent history suggests an ever-growing impact of CEA in the United States, though not as the explicit tool its founders might have imagined. Its application overseas, as discussed in Chapter 8, may foreshadow even greater prospects for the future in the United States.

Clinical Guidelines and Recommendations

The myriad clinical guidelines promulgated by public and private organizations would seem to offer an ideal opportunity for CEA: an area in which the technique could be applied effectively, while remaining below the radar screen. The *Panel on Cost-Effectiveness in Health and Medicine* speculated that practice guidelines issued by medical specialty societies, such as the American College of Physicians, may be a prime target for CEA's influence (Gold et al., 1996, p. 58).

As noted in chapter 3, some evidence suggests that in fact economic analyses are incorporated *in*frequently into clinical guidelines. Wallace and colleagues (2002) reported that few guidelines mention economic analyses in text or references, even when high-quality economic evaluations are available. Yet, even in this study certain types of guidelines were found to incorporate economic information. In particular, guidelines focusing on conditions amenable to risk-factor reduction or preventive care, such as smoking cessation and colorectal cancer screening, were more likely to incorporate economic analyses than, say, surgical therapy for breast cancer.

More important, several major attempts to issue guidelines or recommendations now formally incorporate considerations of cost-effectiveness. The Health Plan Employer Data and Information Set (HEDIS) performance measures for managed-care plans in the United States provide an example.

The National Committee for Quality Assurance (NCQA), the nonprofit organization that established and maintains HEDIS, has recognized the importance of cost-effectiveness as a distinct criterion in selecting new performance measures, noting that measures should "encourage the use of cost-effective activities and/or discourage the use of activities that have low cost-effectiveness" (National Committee for Quality Assurance, 1998). In selecting a measure for a particular clinical condition, NCQA considers cost-effectiveness, as well as other attributes, including the prevalence of the condition and its effect on mortality and morbidity; the availability of effective interventions; the potential for improving the quality of service delivery to enhance the health of the population; and the extent to which the intervention is under the control of the health plan (National Committee for Quality Assurance, 1998).

A recent study found that HEDIS measures do a reasonably good job of reflecting cost-effective practices; that is, most practices covered by HEDIS measures have cost-effectiveness ratios under $50,000/LY or QALY gained, a measure often used as a guide of reasonable value for money (Table 7–1) (Neumann and Levine, 2002). Evidence of cost-effectiveness was available for 11 of the 15 HEDIS measures. For seven of the measures, published evidence indicated that the intervention would be cost-saving and QALY- or LY-increasing for some of the populations covered, though cost-effectiveness ratios varied widely for several of the measures. The range reflects both estimates for different subgroups of populations covered under a measure and varied estimates from different studies for the same population.

Furthermore, U.S. policy makers have begun to incorporate cost-effectiveness information systematically into the development of evidence-based guidelines for health care, including the recent recommendations of the third U.S. Preventive Services Task Force (USPSTF) (Saha et al., 2001), and the Guide to Community Preventive Services (Carande-Kulis et al., 2000).

The consideration of cost-effectiveness in the new USPSTF guidelines is particularly noteworthy because previous incarnations of the Task Force deliberately chose not to incorporate economic information, citing the absence of CEAs for many preventive services, as well as other factors, such as the lack of standards for the field, concerns about the poor quality of existing studies, and fears about explicit rationing (Saha et al., 2001). The latest version of USPSTF justified its use of CEA on several grounds, including the continued rise in health-care costs, theoretical refinements in the field, the promulgation of standards for reporting and conducting CEAs, and a general trend toward better studies (Saha et al., 2001). In developing recommendations today, the USPSTF systematically reviews the cost-effectiveness evidence using a formal data-abstraction tool to help extract useful information and judge the quality of the data to inform its recommendation process. Significantly, the effort endorses the use of cost-utility analyses based on the recommendations of the U.S. Panel on Cost-Effectiveness.

The USPSTF advocates the *selected* use of CEA. The Task Force has noted that the practice would not replace risk-benefit analyses and will not be conducted for every topic, but rather "where relevant questions about cost-effectiveness exist," and where "there are tradeoffs between two or more effective strategies for given health outcomes" (Saha et al., 2001). The Task Force singles out CEA's potential role in understanding the value of various

Table 7–1.   Cost-Effectiveness of Clinical Practices Underlying HEDIS
2000 Measures*

	HEDIS Measure	
	$/QALY: Range	$/LY: Range
PREVENTION OF DISEASE IN ASYMPTOMATIC PERSONS		
Childhood/adolescent immunization status	$1,200–$13,000	Cost-saving – $386,000
Flu shots for older adults		Cost-saving
SCREENING ASYMPTOMATIC PERSONS FOR DISEASE		
Breast cancer screening	%5,100–$19,400	$100–$49,000
Cervical cancer screening	NA	$7,000–$53,000
Chlamydia screening in women	NA	NA
TREATMENT OF PERSONS WITH KNOWN DISEASE TO PREVENT COMPLICATIONS OR RECURRENCES		
Comprehensive diabetes care	Cost-saving – $34,000	Cost-saving – $2,000
Controlling hypertension	$10–$57,000	Cost-saving – $660,000
Antidepressant medication management	Cost-saving – $23,600	NA
Advising smokers to quit	NA	$300–$7,000
Beta-blocker treatment after MI	NA	$3000–$20,000
Cholesterol management after acute cardiovascular events	NA	Cost-saving – $276,000
Use of appropriate medications for asthma	NA	NA
Follow-up after hospitalization for mental illness	NA	NA
MISCELLANEOUS PREVENTIVE MEASURES		
Prenatal care in first trimester	NA	Cost-saving – $2,000
Check-ups after delivery	NA	NA

Source: Neumann and Levine, 2002. Reproduced with permission.

*The cost-effectiveness evidence presented reflects published evidence available as of January 1, 1999. For each HEDIS measure, the published evidence was searched for cost-effectiveness analyses of a similar intervention and target population. Only studies with comparator as "do nothing" or "standard care" were included. $/QALY: dollars per quality-adjusted life year, $/LY: dollars per life year saved. All values expressed in 1998 US dollars and rounded to nearest thousand (except for estimates under $1000).

NA=no published evidence in terms of $/QALY or $/LY available as of Jan. 1, 1999.

screening interval frequencies, or in treating different target populations or risk groups (Saha et al., 2001).

In similar fashion, the *U.S. Guide to Community Preventive Services*, which examines population-based health promotion and disease prevention interventions (e.g., vaccine-preventable disease, motor-vehicle occupancy injury, tobacco use, diabetes prevention, promotion of physical activity), has engaged in a similar process. Investigators for the *Guide* conduct systematic searches and selected economic evaluations, including cost-effectiveness analyses. The researchers abstract data and standardize cost-effectiveness information using specified inclusion criteria (Carande-Kulis et al., 2000).

Medicare

As discussed in chapter 3, Medicare has never incorporated cost-effectiveness analysis formally into its coverage process for new technologies, despite attempts to do so. Nevertheless, cost-effectiveness *has* played a role in isolated coverage decisions, particularly in preventive services (which were not covered when Medicare was created). An example involves coverage of pneumococcal vaccine. In the late 1970s, Congress asked the Office of Technology Assessment to conduct a cost-effectiveness analysis of the vaccine. The study provided a favorable review and played a central role in 1980 legislation permitting Medicare to reimburse for the vaccine (Willems et al., 1980, Warner and Luce, 1982; Schauffler, 1993). Another example involves legislation authorizing Medicare demonstration programs for influenza vaccine, which explicitly stated that services would not be added as permanent benefits unless cost-effectiveness was demonstrated (Schauffler, 1993).[3]

Formal application of CEA has remained for the most part on the sidelines. But this has not stopped federal policy makers from searching for ways to consider value for money in covering new services for Medicare, however. The experience illustrates some important lessons in applying CEA or CEA-like principles in the Medicare program, while avoiding the "third rail" of explicit rationing.

One way involves using terms like "value" and "comparability" rather than "cost-effectiveness." In a carefully crafted Notice of Proposed Rulemaking in 2000 (*U.S. Federal Register*, May 16, 2000), in which the Centers for Medicare and Medicaid Services announced their intention to publish a proposed rule and solicit public comment, the agency outlined how it would consider the comparative health benefits and costs of new technologies for national coverage decisions. Though the rule was never released in proposed or final form, it bears scrutiny as Medicare's attempt to tiptoe around the charged issue of cost-effectiveness while clarifying its "reasonable and necessary" clause and remaining a prudent purchaser of expensive new technology.

First, the Notice categorizes the types of new technologies it will cover:

- A breakthrough technology without consideration of cost;
- A medically beneficial item or service if no other medically beneficial alternative is available;
- A medically beneficial item or service if it is a different clinical modality compared to an existing covered beneficial alternative, without consideration of cost or magnitude of benefit;
- A medically beneficial item or service, even if a less expensive alternative, which is not a Medicare benefit, exists.

Next, the Notice delineates the manner in which CMS will consider evidence: an item must demonstrate both medical benefit and added value:

Step 1: (Medical benefits). Is there sufficient evidence that demonstrates that the item is medically beneficial for a defined population? If no, it is not covered; if yes, then:

Step 2: (Added value). Is there a medically beneficial alternative item or service that is the same clinical modality and is currently covered by Medicare? If no, it is covered; if yes, then:

Step 3. (Added value). Is the item or service substantially more or substantially less beneficial than the Medicare covered alternative? If it is substantially more beneficial (i.e., a breakthrough), it is covered under Medicare. If it is substantially less beneficial, it is not covered under Medicare. If it is deemed equivalent, then:

Step 4 (Added value). Will the item or service result in equivalent or lower costs? If yes, then it is covered under Medicare. If no, then it is not covered.

Note that Step 4 is essentially a cost-minimization determination: if an item or service costs more, but provides no more benefit, it will not be covered. Specifically, the Notice states:

> For clinically substitutable services, it is not reasonable or necessary to pay for incurred costs that exceed the cost of a Medicare-covered alternative that produces the same health outcome. Thus, only by assuring equal or lower costs for the substitutable service could we assure adding value to the pro-

gram. When a service (that is, it has equivalent health outcomes and the same clinical modality) is substantially more expensive than a Medicare-covered alternative would cost considerations lead us to deny coverage for the service. Since we anticipate limiting the application of costs to a narrow situation when two services have equivalent health outcomes and are of the same clinical modality, we need to do only a simple cost-analysis.

The Notice also stated that if a new item or service was equivalent in benefit, was in the same clinical modality, was thus substitutable for the existing service, and was lower in costs, they would consider withdrawing coverage for the more expensive currently covered alternative service. If an item was denied coverage, the requestor could seek more limited coverage targeting a narrower population or submitting new evidence.

CMS never addressed precisely how it would determine whether an item was substantially more or less beneficial, or whether the item will result in equivalent or lower costs, and the Notice solicited comments from the public on the issue.[4] Nor does CMS say how *much* it will pay for items or services that are deemed substantially more beneficial.

Medicare payment policy, a somewhat arcane subject with its own intricacies and experts, is, in fact, seldom discussed in cost-effectiveness circles, though it offers a means of sorts to apply CEA through the back door. Over the years, Medicare has been an innovator in developing payment strategies, creating inpatient and outpatient prospective payment systems, and developing a relative value scale for physician payment, among other advances.

The incentives inherent in any payment system can greatly influence the diffusion of a new medical technology. Prospective payment systems, with fixed payments for each Medicare patient and each DRG based on expected cost of resources in that DRG, create incentives to minimize per-admission treatment costs and to expand admissions in categories where payment exceeds costs. Hospitals also have incentives to move care to uncontrolled settings and to adopt cost-saving technologies even if this has an adverse impact on outcomes or quality, though there are counter-incentives in terms of competition among hospitals and doctors to secure patients by improving quality of care (Garrison and Wilensky, 1986).

How a technology is coded and classified for purposes of Medicare payment can often be as important as the coverage decision itself. For example, an expensive new technology that is assigned to a low-paying DRG provides a disincentive for hospitals to use the product.

On occasion, Medicare officials have noted explicitly that cost-effectiveness could be used to inform *payment* (rather than coverage) decisions, pointing out, for example, that where a technology added nothing new to the ability to diagnose or treat and was also very expensive, Medicare could decide to pay for it at the level of the currently existing technology (Shekar, 1993).

Testifying before the Ways and Means Committee in Congress in 1997, HCFA Administrator Vladeck stated:

> in order to become prudent purchasers of health care, third party payers including HCFA must consider the full value of any medical service they are considering for coverage. Cost-effectiveness analyses, when available, can be used in this regard. These analyses allow us to consider the full range of present and future costs and benefits of a service. Without it, payers and providers often focus on the present costs of expensive technologies rather than on the full value of the service. E.g., if a service is more expensive but equally effective, it would still be covered and paid at the rate of the lower cost alternative. If, however, the service is found to be more effective for a specific group of patients, it could be paid at the higher rate.

Elsewhere in the hearing, he states:

> we have come to the position that even if [a new technology] is no more effective than the preexisting technology, it should be made available in terms of Medicare coverage, but it is not at all clear that we should *pay* the incremental costs unless there is an incremental benefit, and that is the way we are now thinking about these issues. . . . [italics added]

Annual updates to Medicare's prospective payment system are full of implicit considerations about cost-effectiveness. Recent legislation, which includes transitional "pass-through" payments for additional reimbursement for new technology added to the inpatient or outpatient prospective payment systems, also forces the issue.[5] Such payments are made if the technology is new or substantially improved and adds substantially to cost of care in ambulatory payment classification groups or diagnosis-related groups. While regulations raise many questions about how to operationalize the statute (MedPAC, 2001; MedPAC, 2002), and the term "cost-effectiveness" is not used, the law essentially puts Medicare officials in the business of determining which new technologies are cost-effective.

Though Medicare officials deny that they use cost-effectiveness analysis in making coverage decisions, the overall economic impact of a technology seems to influence their decisions. A recent Medicare decision expanded coverage of implantable cardiac defibrillators but stopped short of covering all patients who met the criteria of the pivotal randomized clinical trial. CMS officials denied that they considered cost-effectiveness explicitly, though they did concede the high price tag and budget impact influenced the decision. Steve Phurrough, the acting director of the CMS Coverage and Analysis Group said:

> If an ICD were a buck and a quarter, would we have gone through this entire process of reviewing the evidence at all? Maybe not. But because it's a bit more than a buck and a quarter we wanted to make sure the evidence was clear and that it was a benefit. We don't use cost to decide the evidence issue, but we do use cost to decide if this is important enough to address (O'Riordan, June 13, 2003).

Medicaid

State Medicaid programs, reeling from years of double-digit increases in prescription drug prices and other services, have searched for ways to deliver cost-effective care. Though none has adopted Oregon's prioritization scheme, they have tried other strategies.

States have aggressively promoted generic drugs, developed lists of "preferred" drugs, and implemented cost-sharing payments for high-priced medications (Winslow et al., 2002; Kaiser Commission, 2004). Each policy reflects implicit cost-effectiveness calculations. At a basic level, the promotion of generic drugs reflects a cost-minimization strategy; that is, that the same clinical effect can be obtained for a lower price.

The use of preferred drug lists takes the concept a step further, as states construct lists of therapeutically equivalent products and place lower-priced (and possibly more cost-effective) ones on the favored schedule. The practice forces manufacturers to provide discounts if they want preferred status (Winslow, 2002). Some drug companies have refused to participate in the program, and business groups have questioned the legality of the approach.

The Pharmaceutical Research and Manufacturers Association (PhRMA) has sued on grounds that the provision violates federal Medicaid law by restricting access to drugs and going beyond federally mandated discounts (Winslow et al., 2002). The litigation has turned in part on Medicaid's use of cost-effectiveness information.

The U.S. 11th Circuit Court of Appeals upheld one decision in favor of the Florida Medicaid program to enact a "preferred drug formulary," which exempted certain Medicaid-eligible drugs from prior authorization (U.S. 11th Circuit Court, 2002). Florida Medicaid sought to use a preferred list based on the "clinical, efficacy, safety, and *cost-effectiveness* of a product" (italics added). PhRMA's suit alleged that under the federal statute governing mandated Medicaid drug rebates (42 U.S.C. §1369r-8(d)(4), *clinical factors* (rather than cost-effectiveness) are the only permissible criteria for excluding a drug from the formulary. The court stated that if the Florida law had, in fact, created a Medicaid "formulary," they would agree with PhRMA, because the governing federal statute clearly limits such decisions to clinical issues of safety and effectiveness. The Court found, however, that the Florida law only created a prior authorization program, not a restrictive formulary, and thus did not actually "exclude" any Medicaid-eligible outpatient drug from coverage. Therefore, cost-effectiveness considerations were permissible.

States' use of tiered co-payments (e.g., $15 for a generic drug, $25 for a preferred brand name, and $40 for a non-preferred brand name) have also become popular (Winslow et al., 2002). Determining how to assign a drug to a particular tier turns in theory on considerations of value or cost-effectiveness. It forces a consideration of whether the high-priced, brand-name drug is effective enough to warrant the preferred-tier status.

A few states have begun incorporating cost-effectiveness information explicitly into the process by adopting pharmacoeconomic guidelines for formulary submissions. The guidelines call for evidence-based and value-based considerations for formulary decisions.[6]

Oregon's Medicaid program, for example, was an early and enthusiastic adopter of formulary guidelines. It has contracted out (to investigators at the Oregon Health & Science University in Portland) evidence and cost-effectiveness-based reviews, publicized findings, convened public meetings, and posted analyses on the Internet (Winslow et al., 2002). The Oregon Health Plan's formulary members compare drugs of various classes on the basis of relative effectiveness. To be a preferred drug for the OHP, a drug must be "as effective as any other drug in the class but more cost-effective" (Goldsmith, 2003). In a sense, Oregon, thwarted in its attempt to use cost-effectiveness explicitly and broadly to prioritize health services, has found ways to use cost-effectiveness information in more targeted fashion.

Private Insurers and Managed Care

In a few cases, private insurers and managed-care plans have incorporated cost-effectiveness explicitly into determinations of medical necessity (Jacobsen and Kanna, 2001). Kaiser Permanente, for example, relied on cost-effectiveness analysis in developing guidelines for using contrast agents without resulting litigation (Jacobsen and Kanna, 2001; Eddy, 1992b). The Blue Cross Technology Evaluation Center has provided cost-effectiveness information on a few occasions (Garber, 2001).

Health plans do consider costs in coverage and payment decisions, of course. Indeed, they are obsessed with them. In one recent survey of 346 plans, 90% of medical directors admitted that cost was a factor in decision-making (HCFO, 2003).

For the most part, however, private plans have avoided explicitly using CEA to inform decisions. Instead, they use the information indirectly; that is, to steer patients to low-cost generics; to determine prior authorization; or to influence step-therapy approaches, tiered co-payments, and clinical guidelines (Motheral, 2000; Titlow et al., 2000; Mathematica, 2000; Mohr et al., 2002; Winslow et al., 2002). Considerations of cost-effectiveness may also creep into decisions as medical directors apply the concept of medical necessity to treatment authorization requests (HCFO, 2003).

Health plans also consider costs via "budget impact analyses." They don't combine evidence on effectiveness or cost or confront tradeoffs directly; rather, they pose two separate hurdles: evidence of effectiveness and acceptable budget impact.

Pharmaceutical benefits managers (PBMs), who administer pharmaceutical benefits for health plans and employers, have followed numerous strategies to help their clients. The PBMs process claims, promote formulary compliance, encourage generic substitution, negotiate rebates with manufacturers and retail pharmacies, perform drug utilization review, establish therapeutic exchange and prior authorization programs, administer mail-order deliveries, profile physicians, conduct disease-management programs, maintain lists of preferred drugs, and mobilize pharmacists to urge doctors to switch prescriptions for non-preferred to preferred drugs (Mathematica, 2000). While they aggressively seek cost-effective care, however, they do not seem to have used CEA explicitly as a tool for prioritization.

Instead, day-to-day decisions by plans and PBMs are full of implicit cost-effectiveness calculations. Managers at these organizations are cognizant of this. In one recent survey of formulary decision makers, respondents said that they used pharmacoeconomic information in decisions ranging from formulary drug selection (94% of respondents), development of treatment guidelines (79%), disease management (74%), prior authorization (67%), development of step therapies (62%), and three-tiered copayments (43%) (Motheral et al., 2000). Other surveys have emphasized that concerns about "value" rather than cost as such play a central (though largely unspoken role) in coverage decisions, particularly by the physicians who sit on benefits committees (e.g., Titlow et al., 2000).

Payers in the United States, such as the Veterans' Administration (VA) and the Department of Defense (DoD), have also used cost-effectiveness information to inform formulary decisions. Both the VA and DoD employ closed formularies and maintain low drug prices, which they obtain through aggressive competitive bidding processes for therapeutically interchangeable drugs (Mohr et al., 2002). These payers use their market size (and relative shelter from treacherous political waters) to obtain better prices, by restricting choices of drugs to the least costly alternative if products are therapeutically interchangeable. Coverage decisions follow a policy of medical effectiveness first and cost second—i.e., once a new technology is determined to be effective, cost is considered—including information on "cost-effectiveness, outcomes, cost avoidance" (Mohr et al., 2002; Remund and Valentino, 2003).

Evidence- and Value-Based Formulary Guidelines

Health plans and hospitals have long used drug formularies, which list the prescription medications approved for routine use in the organizations (Dillon, 1999).[7] Yet the process by which these organizations made formulary decisions has frequently lacked transparency or scientific rigor. The pharmacy and therapeutics (P&T) committees overseeing the process have often based decisions on scattered reports in the medical literature, promotional materials provided by drug manufacturers, anecdotal information from physicians, and the extent to which plans could negotiate discounts. To the extent that they conducted their own reviews and analyses, P&T committees tended to focus narrowly on consequences to pharmacy budgets rather than on broader health and economic consequences to the health plan or hospital. In recent years, formulary decision makers have worked to standardize and improve formulary processes, with the goal of grounding decisions in stronger clinical and economic evidence.

The idea of drug formulary committees using explicit value-based evidence guidelines took hold abroad beginning in the early 1990s (see chapter 8). In 1992, Australia became the first country to require drug companies to submit evidence of their product's cost-effectiveness to national authorities as a condition for consideration on the national formulary (Mitchell, 1996). Other countries, including Canada, the United Kingdom, and the Netherlands, followed suit with their own versions (Hjelmgren, 2001).

In the United States, the movement toward formulary guidelines has evolved more slowly. In the absence of any national payer, local plans in the 1980s and 1990s developed internal processes to manage their pharmacy programs, or turned to the growing PBM industry for this service (Navarro and Blackburn, 1999). Formularies became a critical benefit design component.

While formulary committees have used pharmacoeconomic data as an input into their decision-making processes for some time, the information was used informally, and great variation existed among plans (Luce et al., 1996; Titlow et al., 2000; Sloan et al., 1997). With rapid increases in drug spending in the 1990s, health plans and PBMs began to employ formularies more aggressively in an attempt to contain costs. This, combined with the increase in the availability of cost-effectiveness analyses, began to change minds about considerations of value.

In the mid-1990s, U.S. researchers, led by Sean Sullivan of the University of Washington and Paul Langley of the University of Arizona, began developing principles for health plan formulary committees to use pharmacoeconomic evidence in their deliberations (Langley and Sullivan, 1996). Langley and Sullivan (1996) proposed a new format for pharmaceutical submissions to help make health plans' formulary deliberations more evidence-based. The guidelines were adopted by the Regence BlueShield health plan in 1998. Regence began requesting that drug manufacturers submit standardized packages of clinical and economic evidence as a condition of formulary review (Mather et al., 1997; Regence, 2002).

The AMCP Format

In 2000, The Academy of Managed Care Pharmacy (AMCP), a national professional society of pharmacists in managed-care environments, endorsed its own guidelines, based largely on the Regence guidelines, called the AMCP Format for Formulary Submission (hereafter, the "Format"). The organization began encouraging health plans nationwide to implement them (Sullivan et al., 2001; AMCP, 2002).

The Format represents a potential paradigm shift for U.S. formulary committees accustomed to being relatively passive recipients of information submitted by drug companies. It urges health plans to request formally that drug companies present a standardized "dossier," which contains detailed information not only on the drug's effectiveness and safety, but also on its economic value relative to alternative therapies (Table 7–2). The Format further prescribes the layout for the submission, recommending that

Table 7–2.   Information Requested by AMCP Format (Version 2.0)

Item	Description
Product information	• Product description
	• Place of product in therapy
Supporting clinical and economic information	• Summary of key clinical and economic studies
	• Published and unpublished clinical study results
	• Clinical and disease management intervention strategies
	• Outcomes and economic evaluation supporting data
Modeling report	• Model overview
	• Parameter estimates for models
	• Perspective, time horizon and discounting
	• Analyses
	• Presentation of model results
	• Exceptions
Product value and overall cost	
Supporting information	• References contained in dossiers
	• Economic models
	• Formulary submission checklist

Source: Adapted from Academy of Managed Care Pharmacy, "Format for Formulary Submissions: Version 2.0," Academy of Managed Care Pharmacy, Alexandria, VA, October, 2002.

companies include unpublished studies, data on off-label indications, information on the drug's place in therapy, related disease-management strategies, and an economic model that provides evidence of the product's value. While the AMCP guidelines do not represent the first time cost-effectiveness has been considered in formulary decisions, they do mark an important endorsement of the concept and of the idea that standards are needed.

The Format's impact to date

To date, more than 50 health plans, pharmacy benefit management companies, hospitals, Medicaid programs (including Indiana, Kansas, Louisiana, Alabama, Oregon) and other public agencies (e.g., Department of Defense), covering well over 100 million lives, have adopted the Format or a Format-like process (Penna, 2002). The Foundation of Managed Care Pharmacy (FMCP), which oversees research, educational, and other activities for the AMCP has undertaken a series of initiatives to educate pharmacists, pharmaceutical company executives, and other interested professionals about the guidelines (Lyles, 2001).

The advent of formulary guidelines represents a potentially powerful shift for consumers and producers of evidence, and for regulators overseeing the dissemination of promotional material between drug companies and health plans. For health plans and PBMs, guidelines mean more formal internal processes—and the use of cost-effectiveness analysis—for judging evidence. For pharmaceutical companies, the change underscores the importance of differentiating a product's enhanced value relative to alternative therapies. For regulatory authorities, it could signal a profound change in the way they oversee information disseminated by drug companies to health plans. Many critical questions remain, however.

Are formal guidelines better than informal ones?

In theory, one might expect formal guidelines to improve upon informal ones because they promote the use of broader economic and health outcomes to inform decisions, and promise to foster a more careful deliberation about a drug's overall value. Standardized guidelines might enable plans to streamline processes and lower administrative costs.

But these are not foregone conclusions. Whether plans prefer formal guidelines and standards will depend on their costs and benefits in comparison to existing practices. Whether and to what extent explicit guidelines will enhance efficiencies and improve patient care remains unclear and a matter for further evaluation.

Limited empirical evidence is available to date. Awareness of the AMCP Format among health plan managers appears high, though small studies suggest wide variation in plans' adherence to guidelines' recommendations (Jstreetdata, 2001; Robinson et al., 2003), as well as poor quality in submitted materials (Atherly et al., 2001). Data on the guidelines' actual impact on patient outcomes is lacking.

Will formulary guidelines impose an undue burden on health plans and drug companies?

One concern, expressed by health plan and drug company officials anecdotally and in response to small-scale surveys, pertains to the potential burden imposed by new guidelines (Jstreetdata, 2001; Stergachis, 2002; Robinson, 2003).

Such fears are not without foundation. As Sculpher and colleagues (2001) note in commenting on the NICE process, evidence costs money. The AMCP Format asks for resource commitments by both health plans and manufacturers. On the plan side, the Format requires human, technical, and financial resources to support the review process. For manufacturers, the Format means shoring up internal health economics and outcomes research capabilities, or contracting out for preparation of dossiers, which can run up to 100 pages (Cross, 2002).

But there is no reason to believe that guidelines will impose an excessive burden. Over time, efficiencies should develop as plans tinker with the formula and tailor it to their own needs. The Format emphasizes that it is a template rather than a mandate, and that it can be adapted to individual plans (AMCP, 2002).

Plans will probably focus their guideline efforts on big-ticket items or controversial products, such as medications for certain chronic conditions, or expensive innovations like biotechnology injectibles (Jstreetdata, 2001). Because they standardize processes, formulary guidelines may actually reduce the time and resources currently devoted to formulary decision-making (Robinson, 2003).

Ultimately, formulary guidelines are likely to have their greatest impact, not on decisions to accept or reject a drug for formulary, but in guiding questions about its place in therapy: Is it on the preferred drug list? To which subgroups is it targeted? To which formulary tier does it belong?

For their part, drug companies may view guidelines darkly as yet one more hurdle thrown in their path, or more neutrally as a structural change in the marketplace, to which they must adapt. They will also probably see opportunities for showcasing products and for their case on the company's own terms; that is, on the basis of a drug's overall value rather than its acquisition price and negotiated rebates. The changes are likely to accelerate the growth and prominence of health economic and outcomes research divisions (DiMasi et al., 2001). In many ways formulary guidelines represent a continuation of practices they have grown accustomed to overseas, though with a much bigger marketplace and many more players.

Do plans have the expertise?

A concern expressed by drug company officials and some plan managers is that health plans do not have the expertise necessary to judge the information in dossiers, particularly evidence contained in the economic models featured prominently in the guidelines (Stergachis, 2002; Robinson, 2003).

Health plans in the United States, however, are a diverse lot with varied ability to conduct dossier reviews. Some large organizations, such as the Blue Cross and Blue Shield plans or Kaiser, have strong in-house capabilities. Increasingly, Medicaid programs and other payers such as the Department of Defense are developing the expertise or contracting out these services (Otrompke, 2002). Over time other arrangements will undoubtedly evolve. Small plans with insufficient resources will contract with pharmacy benefit management companies (PBMs) for formulary management (Robinson, 2003).

Training efforts will also help. Developing internal capabilities to implement the guidelines involves a steep learning curve, as much as one to two years, according to reports (Jstreetdata, 2001; Robinson, 2003). AMCP has launched a national effort to educate managed-care pharmacy staff in interpreting and integrating data for the formulary review (Lyles, 2001).

Are guidelines a smokescreen for cost-containment?

A larger fear among manufacturers is that plans will employ formulary guidelines as a means to contain costs under the banner of quality improvement.

Though manufacturers may complain that guidelines impose bureaucratic hurdles, impede access to important new drugs, and dampen incentives for innovation (Gorham, 1995; Dent and Sadler, 2002), experience suggests that explicit consideration of evidence tends to increase rather than decrease spending, because it sheds more light on under- rather than over-treatment. In Australia, for example, drug spending grew after the country implemented its pharmacoeconomic guidelines (A. Mitchell, 2002). The NICE process has tended to "level up" access to pharmaceuticals (Taylor, 2001). After Oregon implemented its prioritization scheme, Medicaid expenditures rose faster than those of other Medicaid plans in the country (Leichter, 1999).

Drug companies may not like the hassle and uncertainty that come with new guidelines, but they should not expect a negative impact on overall sales. The larger problem for champions of formulary guidelines will be to handle the expectations of health plan executives, and to convince them that the guidelines are a vehicle to enhance value and not to lower drug expenditures.

Do plans have the clout to force drug companies to comply?

A possible obstacle is that drug manufacturers will refuse to comply with plan requests for information. Drug firms might repudiate demands and instead accelerate traditional promotions aimed at physicians and consumers.

Early experience with the AMCP Format suggests that some companies have balked at providing dossiers, although in the end most have made submissions (Otrompke, 2002). Most likely, drug companies will find obstructionist tactics difficult to sustain. Health plans and PBMs, particularly those with sizable market share, can and will play hardball by insisting on dossiers, and even refusing to review drugs for a formulary if companies do not comply (Otrompke, 2002).

Undoubtedly, problems will persist. Some companies may submit incomplete dossiers, omitting the pharmacoeconomic model, for example, or submitting poor-quality evidence, as has happened abroad (Hill et al., 2000). It may be difficult for plans, particularly small plans, to force companies to comply with all provisions of the Format.

The implementation of formulary guidelines could turn into something of a struggle between big PhRMA versus big managed care, with both sides scoring some early points. However, the AMCP Format gives plans a useful tool for leveling the playing field, which traditionally favored drug manufacturers. Moreover, plans can always threaten to compile dossiers and conduct reviews themselves, or contract them out, if companies refuse to play. They can also put the drug on prior authorization status until a dossier is submitted. In the end, drug companies will probably have no choice but to comply with their customers' requests.

Won't all information submitted by companies be biased?

Another concern is that drug company submissions will be thinly veiled promotional pieces. This fear extends in particular to economic models, whose assumptions are seen as easily manipulated by drug firms.

Such concerns are probably overblown. For one thing companies currently submit information that could be biased. The relevant question is whether the AMCP guidelines will change the potential for bias.

Health plans will naturally expect companies to put their data in the best light possible. They should display a healthy skepticism toward submitted data. Their best defense involves training formulary decision makers about the process and forcing a more honest dialogue.

Moreover, some other safeguards exist. For one, health plans can, as the Format suggests, request full disclosure of funding arrangements between investigators of studies submitted as part of dossiers and the drug companies. For another, dossier submissions must still comply with FDA rules against false or misleading promotion (though how the FDA will regulate such information is a difficult issue).

The U.S. Public Health Establishment

Cost-effectiveness analysis has also found applications—and champions—at other federal health agencies. The Centers for Disease Control and Prevention (CDC) has applied economic models and cost-effectiveness analyses since at least the 1970s. An example was the decision to discontinue routine smallpox vaccination in the United States, and to retain pertussis vaccine in the late 1970s (Corso et al., 2002). Other early work pertained to Legionnaire's disease, folic acid food fortification and supplementation, HIV prevention and treatment, and the prevention of streptococcal infections in newborns (Office of Technology Assessment, 1994).

The CDC today actively employs economic modeling techniques to aid in considerations of disease prevention programs. The Agency maintains a team of some 50 staff economists, decision analysts, and other quantitative experts working on the systematic assessment of the impact of prevention policies and programs (called "prevention effectiveness") (Corso et al., 2002).

A 1999 CDC report emphasized the agency's interest in applying economic evaluation to public health strategies (CDC, 1999). The report outlines strategies for and economic benefits of health promotion and disease and injury prevention in 19 areas of chronic and infectious disease, and injury public health strategies on the basis of health impact, effectiveness, cost of disease or condition, and cost-effectiveness.[8] Each section presents the effectiveness and cost-effectiveness of various prevention strategies.

The Agency for Health Care Research and Quality (AHRQ) (formerly the Agency for Health Care Policy and Research [AHCPR]) has funded scores of projects to examine the costs and outcomes of various health and medical services, and at times has funded methodological work on methods of CEA (Siegel, 2003). The 1992 reauthorization of AHCPR (Public Law 102–410) made two important changes that involved CEA— requiring that individual technology assessments conducted by the Office of Health Technology Assessment must include CEA where valid data existed to support them, and requiring that in producing clinical practice guidelines, AHCPR must consider the cost of alternative medical practices being addressed in the guidelines (OTA, 1994). The National Institutes of Health have also sponsored research on the cost-effectiveness of various services, including the cost-effectiveness of cancer screening and pharmaceutical interventions and use of economic evaluations in clinical trials.

The Office of Management and Budget

The Reagan Administration's Executive Order 12,291, revised in President Clinton's Executive Order 12,866, heralded a coming of age for formal economic evaluation. The Orders affirmed the principle that regulations should be designed in the most cost-effective manner possible, and formally required agencies to prepare a Regulatory Impact Analysis (RIA), including a cost-benefit analysis, for all major federal regulations.[9]

A 2003 OMB report reinforced the philosophy, stating that formal economic analysis can help organize evidence, provide information to determine whether benefits of regulations justify their costs, help discover which alternatives are most cost-effective, and inform the public and other parts of government. It also noted that economic evaluation can show how proposed action is misguided and demonstrate how competing objectives should be balanced with efficiency objectives.

The appointment in 2001 of John Graham as the Administrator of the Office of Information and Regulatory Affairs (OIRA) at the Office of Management and Budget accelerated the importance of economic evaluation and elevated the impact of formal cost-effectiveness analysis. Graham has aggressively sought to use formal cost-effectiveness to identify inconsistencies in government policies toward risk, areas where regulation is inadequate, and existing regulations where costs could exceed any plausible measure of benefits (Hahn, Dudley, 2002).

As examples in 2001, OIRA issued non-binding "prompt letters" from the OMB to government agencies, for example. The first two were sent to the Department of Health and Human Services and the Occupational Safety and Health Administration (OSHA), respectively, asking the agencies to give greater priority to two lifesaving interventions based on cost-effectiveness data—use of automated external defibrillators (AEDs) in the workplace—which data show would be potentially very cost-effective, and the labeling of trans fatty acid content in foods—which data show would avert 2,500 to 5,600 deaths per year with benefits of $25 to $59 billion, while costing $400 to $850 million (U.S. Office of Management and Budget, 2001a; 2001b).

The letter to HHS states that, "In light of these estimates and the recent scientific findings, OMB believes there may be an opportunity here to pursue cost-effective rulemaking that provides significant net benefits to the American people" (OMB, 2001b). The letter to OSHA calls attention to articles in the *Journal of the American Medical Association* and the *New England Journal of Medicine* and other publications on the cost-effectiveness of AEDs (U.S. Office of Management and Budget, 2001a).

According to a press release accompanying the letters, they mark the first time OMB, through OIRA, has publicly used its analytical resources to encourage new regulatory actions as opposed to reviewing decisions initiated by agencies, and are "not meant to have legal authority but rather are designed to bring issues to the attention of agencies in a transparent manner that permits scrutiny and debate" (U.S. Office of Management and Budget, 2001c).

OIRA also made efforts to publicize its actions, opening regulatory debates to a broader audience, employing the Internet, posting documents, and developing an electronic tracking system (Hahn, Dudley, 2002). In early 2002, OIRA listed 23 rules it intends to investigate for potential modification (Hahn, Dudley, 2002).

The 2002 federal budget submission pushes the point further, discussing the usefulness of cost-effectiveness ratios to deploy risk-management resources in a way that achieves the greatest public health improvement for the resources available, in other words, the most "cost-effective" allocation of resources (U.S. Office of Management and Budget, 2002). The budget submission highlights steps the government will take toward the greater use of CEA and league tables in decision making, and also issues government-wide guidelines on information quality to promote greater transparency and consistency in agency analyses of health and safety risks. It also notes that the OMB has committed to updating periodically its guidelines for regulatory analyses used when the OMB reviews agency rulemakings, and encouraging agencies to develop objective measures of program effectiveness to facilitate cost-effectiveness analyses (U.S. Office of Management and Budget, 2002).

In a subsequent report to Congress on the costs and benefits of major health and safety regulations,[10] OMB called for improving the technical quality of benefit-cost estimates, and expanding methods to embrace cost-effectiveness analysis as well as cost-benefit analysis in regulatory analyses. The report, which provided cost-effectiveness estimates for selected interventions (Table 7–3), shows how far the methodology has come.

While this report does not favor cost-effectiveness analysis over cost-benefit analysis, it does encourage agencies to do both because they offer somewhat different, but useful, perspectives. It calls for more uniform analytical guidance and increased transparency in analyses, as well as for certain changes and innovations. For example, it states that agencies should report estimates using several discount rates, and that agencies should employ formal probability analysis of benefits and costs for rules that will have more than a $1 billion-impact on the economy (Draft 2003 Report

Table 7–3.   Cost per Life-Year Saved for Selected Interventions

Intervention or Regulation	Type	Cost per Life-Year Saved (US$2001)
Petroleum Refining NESHAP (EPA)	Health	Cost-saving (<0)
Powered Industrial Truck Operating Training (OSHA)	Safety	Cost-saving (<0)
Head Impact Protection (DOT)	Safety	$50,000–53,000
Reflective Devices for Heavy Trucks (DOT)	Safety	$69,000
Child Restraints (DOT)	Safety	$105,000–331,000
Rail Roadway Workers (DOT)	Safety	$523,000
Interim Enhanced Surface Water Treatment (EPA)	Health	<0 to $679,000
NOx SIP Call (EPA)	Health	$373,000–714,000
Methylene Chloride (OSHA)	Health	$1.16 million
Stage I Disinfection By-Products (EPA)	Health	<0 to infinite

Source: Federal Budget Submission, 2003. Technical details to be found at www.whitehouse.gov/omb. EPA = Environmental Protection Agency. OSHA = Occupational Safety and Health Administration. DOT = Department of Transportation. NESHAP = National Emissions Standards for Hazardous Air Pollutants.

to Congress, Appendix C. OMB Draft Guidelines for the Conduct of Regulatory Analysis and the Format of Accounting Statement). The report also underlines problems with the approach: that cost-effectiveness results based on averages need to be treated with great care, and that CEA can be misleading when the effectiveness measure does not weight appropriately the consequences of each alternative. The OMB goes onto ask for actual underlying data—mortality and morbidity, age distribution of affected population, severity and duration of disease conditions or trauma, etc.—so OMB can make apples to apples comparisons. It also requests separate description of distributional effects, authorized by EO12866, and notes that even if difficult to quantify this should provide relevant information and identify quantifiable effects.

8

Cost-Effectiveness Analysis Abroad

. . . .

> *NICE offers the NHS and its patients a new service, which we intend*
> *shall earn, and retain, the confidence and respect of the community as a*
> *whole.*
> —Professor Sir Michael Rawlins, Chair, National Institute
> for Clinical Excellence

The International Community and Priority-Setting in Health Care

The international experience in using cost-effectiveness information to explicitly inform formulary decisions provides a remarkable contrast to that of the United States. For a number of years, the United Kingdom, Canada, Australia, and other countries have incorporated cost-effectiveness considerations explicitly into processes for making coverage and pricing decisions about drugs and other technologies (e.g., Laupacis, 2002; Mitchell, 2002; Hjelmgren et al., 2001).

Unlike the United States, where there has been little public acknowledgment of limits to health resources, a number of European countries (including Norway, Denmark, Sweden, and the Netherlands) established national commissions in the 1980s and 1990s to discuss priorities and choices and to create an explicit framework for limit-setting.

While these commissions elicited controversy, they were also greeted by public discussions and broad-based support of the need for a limit-setting process. Daniels and Sabin (2002) call these early efforts the first points on the social learning curve. A 1987 Norwegian report urged that priorities be set by ranking programs or interventions on one of five levels, depending on the seriousness of the disease or condition. The first tier gives priority to interventions deemed necessary because of imminent risk to lives of individuals or groups—emergency medicine; the second to interventions to address diseases with catastrophic but not imminent consequences; the third to interventions where consequences we not as serious; the fourth to those improving health and quality of life but consequences less significant; the fifth to those not necessary or supported only with ambiguous evidence. But the approach did not take into account the degree of effectiveness of a treatment or cost. A report from the Netherlands gave considerations of efficiency or cost-effectiveness an important role in its deliberations but alongside other factors. The report asked four questions:

(1) Is it necessary care from the community point of view? (2) Is it demonstrated to be effective? (3) Is it efficient? (4) Can it be left to individual responsibility?

Daniels and Sabin (2002) note that other nations have addressed problems of scarcity in different ways, though there have been several important experiences for cross-national learning: discussion centered on what constitutes fair process, need for transparency, community involvement, and a mechanism for encouraging deliberation in the broader democratic process, transparent tools, grappling with the role of experts and how much openness is desirable, appeals process, and convergence in diverse countries on how to ration fairly and establish legitimacy.

In recent years, many countries have issued voluntary or mandatory pharmacoeconomic guidelines (Hjelmgren et al., 2001; Akehurst, 2001). These include Denmark, Finland, France, Hungary, Ireland, Italy, the New Zealand, Netherlands, Norway, Portugal, Spain, Switzerland, and the United Kingdom. The various guidelines share many similarities. All reflect attempts to standardize the clinical and economic information on new drugs (and in some cases other technologies) presented to healthcare decision makers. For example, guidelines typically spell out the methodological and reporting requirements—such as the analysis framework and the types of costs and health outcomes to be estimated and reported. Sometimes, they specify the particular types of analysis desired (e.g., cost-utility analysis), as well as the perspective expected (e.g., societal or National Health Service). Guidelines also tend to specify or suggest the format for modeling, time horizon, discounting, sensitivity analyses, and the presentation of results. Finally, they often ask for "financial impact" or "budget impact" analyses.

Some differences exist among guidelines, namely in the choice of perspective or resources to be included (Hjelmgren et al., 2001). For example, while most guidelines prefer a societal perspective, some ask for direct costs only, while others also request information on indirect costs. Four examples—from Australia, the United Kingdom, Canada, and the World Health Organization (WHO)—are reviewed here to illustrate the opportunities and challenges inherent in such policies.

Australia

In 1992, Australia announced that it would require drug companies to submit evidence on the comparative cost-effectiveness of new pharmaceuticals before listing them on the national formulary, and that it would use the information to guide decisions on reimbursing new products (Mitchell, 2002). Since then, no new drug can be listed on national formulary (the Australian Pharmaceutical Benefits Scheme) as a pharmaceutical benefit unless the Pharmaceutical Benefits Advisory Committee (PBAC), an independent, statutory body, makes such a recommendation to the Minister of Health. The PBAC is required by law to consider the effectiveness and cost of a proposed benefit compared to alternative therapies.[1]

The pharmacoeconomic guidelines have been through several revisions; Australia is currently working on the third revision (Mitchell, 1996 & 2002). In addition, the cost-effectiveness criteria have been applied for different health care interventions over the years in Australia: pharmaceuticals in 1991; services, procedures, and diagnostics in 1997; vaccines in 1997; blood products in 1998; population health in 1999; and screening programs on ad hoc basis throughout. In implementing its policy, Australia argued that cost-effectiveness was relevant to price—if a new drug offered more benefit than current alternatives, it should be rewarded with a higher price—and that cost-effectiveness is an extension of the larger movement toward evidence-based medicine (Mitchell, 2002).

A drug can be listed as eligible to be subsidized in Australia after two steps: (1) it is recommended by the Pharmaceutical Benefits Advisory Committee; (2) following a positive recommendation by PBAC, the drug is then declared by the Minister of Health to be a pharmaceutical benefit and thus listed on the national formulary. Thus, if there is no positive recommendation by the PBAC, the minister cannot add the drug.

The pharmaceutical company makes a submission and lists a price. The PBAC then has two bases for recommendations. One is a listing based on cost-minimization, where there is insufficient health reason to justify a higher price over the main comparator. The case may default to a cost-minimization analysis (which assume that outcomes of two treatments are equal) if two trials are done on separate drugs, both with the same common reference (e.g., placebo). "Me-too" drugs typically don't receive a higher price, though there have been concerns about the true equivalence of products categorized in the same therapeutic class, and some exceptions have been made, such as for H2 receptor antagonists, ACE inhibitors, some calcium channel blockers, and some statins (Mitchell, August 2002, personal communication). The policy on me-too drugs' not receiving a premium price holds even if a therapeutic class includes a generic alternative. That is, the brand-name product is held to the generic drug price in the class.

The PBAC can also base its recommendation on acceptable *cost-effectiveness* evidence. This criterion applies when authorities deem a new drug to represent a true health advance. The innovator is rewarded with a higher price. Health officials judge the strength of the evidence to determine whether or not the PBAC should grant a premium price.

If the PBAC decides that a premium price for an innovative new drug is *not* justified by the accepted health advantage, it may consider two policy levers before resorting to rejection, and, according to officials, both are explored simultaneously, to see where it might be acceptably cost-effective. One level involves reducing the *price* to one that makes the drug cost-effective. The other is to restrict use of the drug to subgroups of patients likely to benefit the most. More often than not, authorities use the subgroup lever over the price lever (Mitchell, personal communication, August 2000). One key related issue involves how much "leakage" there is outside the restriction placed on appropriate subgroups for prescribing.[2]

Typically, there are 80 to 100 submissions per year, of which approximately one-third are resubmissions. The PBAC employs about 50 people and also contracts work to external groups. In addition, there is another government branch involved in setting and enforcing restrictions. A new policy requires a cabinet-level decision for any drug that will have an impact of more than $10 million (AUS).

Problems have been reported with the quality of drug company submissions, mostly related to poorly supported inferences from the clinical data available (see Hill et al., 2000). In terms of the Australian policy's overall impact, evidence is limited. George et al. (2001) recently found that decisions to recommend drugs for listing by the PBAC were generally consistent with cost-effectiveness evidence. The authors reviewed 35 CEAs submitted to the PBAC between January 1991 and June 1996 (26 cost-effectiveness analyses and 9 cost-utility analyses) and reported a significant difference between the C/E ratios for drugs recommended for listing and those not. The PBAC was unlikely to recommend a drug if the cost-effectiveness ratio exceeded $76,000 per life year (AUS) and unlikely to reject if the ratio was less than $42,000/LY, though the authors note that CUAs represented only 8% of all submissions during this time.

NICE

With the establishment of the National Institute for Clinical Excellence (NICE) as a Special Health Authority in the Department of Health for England and Wales in April 1999, the United Kingdom brought the active use of cost-effectiveness to one of Europe's largest markets.

NICE emerged as part of the new Labour government's health policy in the 1990s but had its roots in the growing evidence-based medicine movement and in long-standing concerns about access and health costs in the United Kingdom (Raferty, 2001; Drummond, 2001; Akehurst, 2001). The desire to eliminate ineffective treatments was highlighted by "postcode prescribing," a term used to describe wide, unexplained regional variations in the use of medications. NICE's creation was also spurred by a large and vocal cadre of health economists in the country, who for decades had promoted CEA as a way to optimize available budgets (Akehurst, 2001).

The stated mission of NICE is "to provide patients, health professionals and the public with authoritative, robust and reliable guidance on current best practise" (National Institute of Clinical Excellence, 2003). Its mandate is to examine the "broad balance of benefits and costs" as well as "the degree of clinical need of the patients with the conditions under consideration."

NICE issues nonbinding guidance to the National Health Service on both individual health technologies (including drugs, medical devices, diagnostic techniques, and medical and surgical procedures) and the clinical management of specific conditions. With 30 staff members and a 10-million-pound budget, and relying heavily on external consultants at seven academic centers across the United Kingdom, NICE has been called a "virtual organization" (Raferty, 2001).

Unlike the case in Australia, where drug companies must demonstrate cost-effectiveness before a listing for reimbursement, NICE issues a call for appraisal itself. Topics are referred to NICE by a special "horizon scanning group." Members of the public can suggest that a certain technology or clinical topic be referred to NICE. Also, in contrast to Australia, the United Kingdom has no restricted national formulary of medicines. NICE guidance is issued in order to disseminate information on the effectiveness and cost-effectiveness of key services to the medical community (Drummond, 2001).

In reviewing a technology, NICE considers the quality of evidence, including effectiveness and cost-effectiveness, as well as the degree of uncertainty and the existence of alternative treatment. Cost-effectiveness issues inform, but are not the sole determinants of, the Institute's guidance. NICE's mandate also states that it will consider factors such as equity of opportunity, impact on innovation, and the budget impact of a service to the NHS. Final decisions include considerations about whether the technology is supported at all, which patient groups are the best candidates, and when to start and stop treatment.

The United Kingdom's Treasury Department monitors NICE's decisions to determine implications of health care appraisals for total expenditures. If a technology meets NICE appraisal criteria but is unaffordable with the resources available, Parliament, not the Institute itself, decides on actual resource allocation. NICE's provisional decisions are issued before final ones are made, and interested parties have the right to appeal. According to one estimate, NICE's recommendations to use technologies have increased costs to the NHS by £575 million through mid-2002 (Mayor, 2002).

NICE has worked to make its process transparent and to involve input from stakeholders. The Institute publishes appraisals on its website at several stages: scope of appraisal, literature review, provisional views, and draft guidance. Meetings are held with all stakeholder groups, including relevant patient organizations, doctors, and pharmaceutical companies (Mayor, 2002). A first meeting of a citizens' council took place in the fall of 2002, and according to reports, 4500 people applied for 30 places for non-medical representatives of the general public (Mayor, 2002).

Impact to date

Since its inception, NICE's actions, and particularly its application of cost-effectiveness analysis, have elicited strong reactions. NICE's very first recommendation, advising physicians not to prescribe zanamivir during the 1999/2000 influenza season because it was perceived as having excessive costs relative to any expected benefits obtained, was highly controversial and set the tone for the criticism to follow.

NICE has been praised and faulted on various grounds. Some have criticized as cumbersome the strategy of considering one intervention at a time, rather than using an Oregon-like system, which would consider all services at once (Smith, 2000). Critics point to the impossibility of a single national committee's tackling more than a fraction of the questions that patients and doctors need answered (Lipman, 2001).

NICE has been criticized for being an instrument of rationing care (and "unfortunately," remarked one observer, "it's not a very good one" (Smith, 2000)). Some have charged that the process delays access to life-saving treatments such as Herceptin for the treatment of metastatic breast cancer (Burke, 2002). Others have claimed that the agency has ignored its mandate to encourage innovation (Dent and Sadler, 2002), and has been overly bureaucratic (Lipman, 2001). Some have argued that rather than encouraging evidence-based medicine, it imposes a top-down "one size fits all" population view of medicine (Lipman, 2001).[3] Smith called it a recipe for unjust rationing by delay, discrimination, dilution, and diversion. Reports suggest that the pharmaceutical industry has generally been hostile, though perhaps with signs of increasing engagement over time (Raferty, 2001).

NICE's openness and transparency have been praised in other quarters. For example, observers point to NICE's practice of publishing provisional and final appraisals on its website (Raferty, 2001; Sculpher et al., 2001). The case of imatinib (Gleevec) for the treatment of chronic myeloid leukemia (CML) illustrates the potential for NICE flexibility. The Institute first recommended the drug only for patients in the accelerated phase of the disease, but then changed the recommended indication for patients in the chronic or blast crisis phase as well, if interferon alpha had failed or could not be tolerated (Mayor, 2002).

There have been complaints that the actual bases for final decisions are unclear, specifically that it is difficult to determine whether input from consumer groups is actually taken into account, whether quality-of-life evidence truly matters, and whether there exists a "hard" cost-effectiveness threshold above which NICE rejects technologies (Kmietowicz, 2001; Dent and Sadler, 2002). The editor of *BMJ* has argued that far from being transparent, the process is driven by political clout as much as by evidence (Smith, 2000). Critics have also questioned NICE's independence from drug companies and politicians (e.g., Smith, 2000; Howell, 2001; Walker, 2001; Burke, 2002).

Specific decisions have come under fire, particularly with respect to zanamivir (Powell, 2001), but also for cholinesterase inhibitors for Alzheimer's disease (Dent and Sadler, 2002), implantable defibrillators (Burke, 2002), and the use of interferon beta and glatiramer acetate for multiple sclerosis (Ellis, 2001).

How much impact NICE has had is not entirely clear. The organization can fulfill its promise only if its guidance is implemented by a national health service that supports the changes NICE promotes (Dent and Sadler, 2002). Health authorities in the United Kingdom have said on occasion that they have no cash to implement NICE guidelines and that other government priorities make it difficult to implement NICE requirements, though Prime Minister Blair has repeatedly promised new money for the system (Burke, 2002).

NICE has also been criticized for an inability to say no, except in obvious cases (Smith, 2000; Raferty, 2001; Burke, 2002). Some evidence supports this contention: of the first 22 health technologies it considered up to March 2001, NICE recommended *against* in only three cases (prophylactic removal of wisdom teeth, laparoscopic surgery for colorectal cancer; and autologous cartilage transplantation for defects in knee joints) (Raferty, 2001). (Zanamivir was not recommended but the decision was later reversed.)

There has been lively debate about whether a cost-effectiveness "threshold" exists above which NICE won't recommend services. NICE claims officially that the agency doesn't maintain a strict threshold, though its chairman seems to have suggested that one exists (Devlin, 2002).[4] An upper threshold of about £30,000/QALY seems to have emerged (Taylor, 2001). Though cost per QALY ratios have been cited in only one-half of NICE's recommendations, the Institute's recommendations (including recommendations on restricting the use of a particular drug or device) have roughly been consistent with this threshold (Table 8–1) (Raferty, 2001; Towse and Pritchard, 2002).

Towse and Pritchard (2002) point to NICE's decision on the anti-obesity drug orlistat, in which a very explicit reference was made to a £20–30,000 threshold. The NICE report stated, "to attain a sufficient level of cost-effectiveness, in the region of a cost per QALY gained of between £20–30K, people treated with orlistat (Xenical) have to lose about 5% of body mass for each of three months that they are maintained on treatment, or achieve a cumulative loss of at least 10% of body weight from the start of treatment

Table 8–1.   NICE Decisions by Cost-Effectiveness Threshold, 1999–2003.

Cost per QALY (in £)	Accepted	Restricted	Rejected
< 20	36	11	4
20–30	8	7	2
> 30	4	8	11

Source: Towse and Pritchard, 2002; C. Pritchard, personal communication, January, 2004.

X2 = 9.8, p<0.05, but sensitive to life year to QALY conversion over the first six months." The NICE Appraisal committee subsequently recommended that orlistat should be available for those who meet this weight reduction criterion.

In addition, a U.K. Department of Health circular noted that high (i.e., unfavorable) cost/QALY estimates for technologies have only been accepted if there were "*special factors* . . . not covered by the formal modeling" [italics added] (Towse and Pritchard, 2002).

What, then, are these special factors? NICE has recommended technologies that exceeded the £30K/LY threshold in a few cases, such as riluzole for motor neuron disease (only amyotrophic lateral sclerosis) with an estimated C/E ratio of £34 to £44K, and beta interferon or glatiramer acetate for MS, which NICE first rejected but later overturned (Raferty, 2001; Towse and Pritchard, 2002). The recommendation for riluzole cited "the severity and relatively short life span of people with ALS and in particular . . . the values which patients place on the extension of tracheotomy free survival time" (Raferty, 2001; NICE, 2003b).

The NICE decision on drugs for multiple sclerosis has attracted a great deal of attention. Debates in part have involved technical details of the models underlying cost-effectiveness estimates, particularly how to judge long-term efficacy based on the limited available short-term clinical trials. The issue also provoked strong reactions from patient advocates and politicians on moral grounds (Taylor, 2001). NICE provided a conditional recommendation in favor of the multiple sclerosis (MS) drugs despite evidence showing unfavorable cost-effectiveness ratios: at least an order of magnitude higher than the £30,000/QALY standard (Taylor, 2001). However, the decision involved a "conditional coverage" that allows the government to share risk; if there is no improvement in patients, drug companies must pay the cost. Essentially, NICE established an outcomes guarantee for pharmaceuticals (S. Chapman, 2003), whereby the drug company and prescribing stakeholders agree on outcomes expected from drugs in a given indication. If the drug fails to fulfill expectations, the pharmaceutical company refunds the health service for the cost of the drug.

The existence of NICE may also have the effect of restricting U.K. drug prices, since drug companies keep the £30K threshold in mind when pricing a drug for the U.K. market (Taylor, 2001; Towse, personal communication, September 2002). But there are other layers of control that can affect drug prices, including generally tight prescribing budgets at the physician practice and primary care level (Adrian Towse, personal communication) and an explicit profit control mechanism, based on return on capital, whereby companies submit data to the Department of Health and, according to internal formulas, grant a rebate or reduce the price of their drug if they exceed the targeted rate. Also, for drugs used on an inpatient basis, a hospital drug and therapeutics committee has additional negotiating power because they, unlike those who treat outpatients, have power to limit the number of drugs on formulary.

Canada

Canada's experience with cost-effectiveness analysis has its roots in the late 1980s with the establishment of the Canadian Coordinating Office for Health Technology Assessment (CCOHTA), as a national voice for health technology assessment (CCOHTA, 2003). CCOHTA functions as an independent body at arm's length from the government to give regional and local authorities information on the clinical effectiveness and cost-effectiveness to inform decisions for Canada's publicly funded health-care system. In 2002, CCHOTA's mandate expanded to include management of common review process for new drugs submitted to participating federal provincial and territorial drug benefit programs.

The move to use formal pharmacoeconomic guidelines began in Ontario in the mid-1990s. Today, a Drug Quality and Therapeutics Committee of Ontario Ministry of Health recommends to the Health Minister which drugs should be included in the drug benefit program for individuals over the age of 65 (Laupacis, 2002). The Ministry rarely rejects the Committee's recommendation. The Therapeutics Committee contains 10 physicians and two pharmacists, whose members serve three to five years. Companies that wish to have a drug on the formulary prepare a detailed submission using a checklist describing clinical and cost-effectiveness. The submissions are reviewed by external consultants who assume a societal perspective in making recommendations. The Committee, where a simple majority rules, may approve drugs for general benefit, limited use, or use only under specific requests sent to the Drug Programs Branch of the Health Ministry.

As in other countries, the process has engendered debate (Laupacis, 2002). Industry has viewed the approach as a cost-containment exercise rather than one to establish value. Members of the public and private arena have complained that they have no input into the process. The deliberations of the Committee are confidential, though if a drug is not listed, the company receives a written summary and may appeal.

The actual impact of the program remains unclear. Despite complaints about the program's restrictiveness, drug spending continues to rise rapidly. Andreas Laupacis, a long-time expert in cost-effectiveness analysis and a member of the Committee, recently observed that cost-effectiveness decisions tend to be determined by effectiveness rather than by costs, and that subtleties in the cost-effectiveness methodology usually do not play a role in final decisions. He has also written that "Although the Therapeutics Committee does not use an explicit threshold for what is cost-effective, my sense is that the committee's threshold is different from that suggested in our article, for example, $50,000 per quality adjusted life year would be considered relatively unattractive" (Laupacis, 2002).

The Committee has been quite willing to recommend against listing. In 1999/2000, for example, recommendations for nongeneric drugs were divided as follows: (1) general benefit (11%), (2) limited use (27%), and (3) Section 8 (62%) (Section 8 involves a specific request sent to the Drug Programs Branch of the Ministry of Health and Long Term Care, where the request is reviewed by ministry staff and a decision about reimbursement made (Laupacis, 2002). The reasons why a drug does not receive a General Benefit listing include: effectiveness compared to available therapies is small; a drug's price is higher than that of the most frequently used comparator drug but it is only marginally more effective; the drug's effectiveness is not convincingly demonstrated (e.g., there are no head-to-head trials); the drug is only cost-effective in a particular subgroups of patients (Laupacis, 2002).

Studies have traced problems in the quality of submissions and in general have found poor compliance with recommendations for good CEA practices, especially with industry-funded studies. Anis and Gagnon, (2000), for example, reviewed all submissions with economic analyses (n = 88) to the British Columbia drug plan between January 1996 and April 1999: 25 cost-consequences analyses; 14 CEAs; 11 cost-minimization analyses; nine CUAs or cost-benefit analyses; 29 budget impact analyses. They found that 45% used an inappropriate comparator, 61% lacked sensitivity analysis, and there were many problems with elements such as the study perspective and time horizon. Of the total, 74% of submissions were not recommended for listing, 16% were approved for restricted benefit; and 9% as full benefit. Submissions with CEAs that adhered to guideline recommendations were more likely to be recommended for reimbursement.

The World Health Organization (WHO) and the Developing World

In 1998, given the paucity of cost-effectiveness analysis in low- and middle-income countries, and the wide range over which the physical infrastructure, human resources, and political considerations varied enormously across countries and regions, the World Health Organization launched an ambitious initiative called the WHO-CHOICE (Choosing Interventions that are Cost-Effective) program to provide decision makers with evidence for priority-setting to help improve the performance of health systems (World Health Organization, 2003). The objective was to develop standardized methods for cost-effectiveness analysis that can be applied to all interventions.

This program is assembling regional databases for 17 geographical areas grouped on the basis of epidemiology, infrastructure, and economic situation. The data will cover the costs, impact on population health, and cost-effectiveness of a wide range of health interventions using standardized methodology, and summarizing the results in regional databases available on the Internet. Thus far, the work has focused on seven areas: unsafe water, sanitation, and hygiene; addictive substances; childhood malnutrition; other nutrition-related risk factors and physical inactivity; sexual and reproductive health; unsafe injections; and iron deficiency. The idea is to provide information that would allow analysts to adjust the results of regional databases to their country, and give them a menu of interventions that are cost-effective in each region, a list of those that are not cost-effective, and another set of interventions in between.

Conclusion

Other countries' use of CEA underscores the fact that the United States's failure to use the approach is driven more by its own cultural, political, and institutional conditions, rather than by the technique's inherent methodological shortcomings.

The experiences abroad shows that using CEA requires political will from politicians and policy makers. It also illustrates that it is difficult to separate use of CEA information from the systems in which it is being used. Many of the charges leveled at the use of CEA abroad are in fact attacks against the effects of centralized decision-making and the lack of market incentives, rather than indictments of cost-effectiveness analysis per se.

But other countries have shown that, at its best, CEA can focus debate on the overall value of a technology or program rather than its acquisition or implementation cost. It can help guide scarce resources towards their most efficient uses. The challenge is how to incorporate these advantages of CEA in the pluralistic U.S. health care system.

9

Imagining a Future for CEA

. . . .

*We are at beginning of a long learning curve since the problem of meeting
diverse needs fairly under resource constraints is an unsolved problem of
distributive justice that societies have just begun to address.*

—Norman Daniels and James Sabin, 2002

What Have We Learned in 25 Years?

Reassessing CEA's impact in the United States

After 25 years of cost-effectiveness analysis in health and medicine, it is a
good time to reassess its impact. Has cost-effectiveness analysis had any
influence?

The short answer is "Of course." Cost-effectiveness analyses have become a ubiquitous presence in health and medical journals and an important component of evidence-based medicine. By its sheer existence, CEA
changes the nature of conversations about the impact of investments in health
care. It forces and focuses discussions about the value of health and medical services within a clear theoretical framework. The thousands of articles
in the peer-reviewed literature over the years attest to its currency among
researchers and thought leaders. It exerts an influence over decisions large
and small: of formulary committees, technology assessment panels, guideline developers, and public health agencies.

At the same time, it has fallen short of expectations. The vision of proponents who wanted to use CEA as a formal tool for prioritizing health
services never materialized. Explicit use of CEA was discarded, even in
Oregon, the only payer in the U.S. to rally to its cause. Even less restrictive

forms of cost-effectiveness analysis have not been incorporated formally into policy-making. Medicare abandoned its efforts to include cost-effectiveness as a criterion for covering new technologies. Private health plans have generally avoided it. A generation after its appearance in the medical literature, champions of the technique must feel at least somewhat disappointed about its track record.

While always acknowledging that CEA was only one input into healthcare decisions, proponents failed to predict the unwillingness or inability of policy makers in the United States to apply the tool explicitly. After considering the potential political fallout, most public and private industry officials have shied away from its use.

An important lesson is that using cost-effectiveness ratios to make mechanical rankings is unacceptable. In retrospect, this shortcoming seems obvious. The medical community was forewarned. Champions of the technique have long cautioned against using ratios rigidly.

Still, applying cost-effectiveness ratios to "solve" resource allocation problems was always the goal. Why painstakingly estimate cost-effectiveness ratios unless they could be used? The field has never really addressed the dissonance this created. The *Panel* simultaneously stated that the greater part of the decision-making process lies outside of the cost per QALY ratio (Gold et al., 1996, p. 12), while claiming that "the larger the number of cost-effectiveness analyses that include a reference case, the larger the number of meaningful comparisons" (Gold et al., 1996, p. xxi). The field's roots in engineering and operations management have always held the allure that investments in health care could be treated as optimization problems. To create a highly structured instrument and then claim that it should not be used too literally is at best unhelpful. The backers of the Oregon plan were simply following the principles of cost-effectiveness analysis to their natural endpoints. We now appreciate that Oregon-like solutions do not provide practical models.

A second lesson is that it is difficult to use cost-effectiveness analysis in less restrictive fashion. Public and private insurers, for example, have not been willing to use cost-effectiveness even as one of several criteria for covering new medical services.

What does this auger for the future? Despite setbacks, excessive pessimism about the prospects of CEA would be misplaced, too. CEA has found a permanent place on the health policy landscape and will undoubtedly endure. Still, the community needs a better understanding of its role and its limitations.

Acceptable uses of CEA

What then *is* acceptable when it comes to CEA in the United States?

First, the acceptability of publishing cost-effectiveness analysis in main-stream American medical journals represents an important development. The methodology has gained a permanent foothold. A published cost-effectiveness ratio is a powerful focal point for debates. Researchers will continue to investigate the value of medical and public health interventions. Drug and device companies will continue to provide evidence that their products offer good value despite high price tags.

Beyond that, U.S. policy makers have gravitated toward a policy of "cost-effectiveness once removed." The emerging rules of engagement allow decision makers to consider cost-effectiveness analysis, but only at arm's length, avoiding the perception that they are explicitly rationing resources.

In practice, this means that clinicians and insurers can use CEA indirectly by appealing to clinical guidelines that incorporate them. CEAs can and have influenced guidelines about the optimal ages at which to begin or to stop treatment, the frequency with which to screen for a particular disease, or the lab values that trigger a workup (Eddy 1992c; Wallace et al., 2002).

Medicare can also use cost-effectiveness analysis at a distance. It can use analyses to inform payment decisions such as deciding not to pay more for an expensive technology that doesn't offer substantial benefits compared to an existing alternative.

In this manner, rationing under the radar is permitted. Payers maintain their reputations and some measure of protection against lawsuits. Patients safeguard their trust in their doctors. Physicians preserve the impression that their patients' interests are paramount, and that a sense of fairness pervades, even while understanding at some level their role in apportioning scarce societal resources.

This desire for breathing space means that guidelines incorporating cost-effectiveness are more palatable when they involve broad public health and preventive services rather than acute care treatments. Researchers have already found some empirical basis for this. In their review of guidelines' use of cost-effectiveness analysis, Wallace et al. (2002) reported that conditions amenable to preventive care, such as smoking cessation and cancer screening strategies, were more likely to incorporate economic analyses than surgical therapies. The authors suggested that there might be a stronger rationale to justify program benefits economically when benefits will occur in the future compared to treatments with more immediate impact.

It is also consistent with the recent consideration of CEA by the U.S. Preventive Services Task Force (USPSTF). Notably, the USPSTF singled out CEA as particularly useful for determining optimal interventions for screening and the different target populations or risk groups who might be suitable for preventive services (Saha et al., 2001). Moreover, the USPSTF emphasized that it would not create rankings of cost-effectiveness ratios for preventive services, and that it would use CEA only in selective cases (Saha et al., 2001).

The Way Forward

Imagining a future for cost-effectiveness analysis

One scholar of the field recently observed that "cost-effectiveness analysis has had, at best, a troubled youth . . . but it will give way to a successful adulthood" (Ubel, 2000, p 173). He goes on to predict that administrators, policy makers, and others will become more adept at using CEA.

But how to get there?

Some have called for a broad cultural shift in the way society thinks about resource allocation and cost-effectiveness analysis (e.g., Powers and Eisenberg, 1999; Prosser et al., 2000; Weinstein, 2001). Accordingly, this would involve persuading practicing physicians to embrace CEA more openly. Physicians may be in the best position to use CEA effectively, in that unlike the case with higher-level forms of rationing (e.g., by formulary committees or utilization reviewers), physicians at the bedside can consider the case of specific patients and take into account their individual charac- teristics and preferences (Ubel, 2000, pp. 99–100, 124). A body of opinion in professional and lay literature supports rationing by doctors as neces- sary and ethical, and that masking it erodes the trust and moral standing of physicians (Levinsky, 1998).

The need for greater *public* awareness and debate on the tension be- tween what is medically possible and what is affordable has also been emphasized (Sacramento Health Care, 2001). Weinstein (2001) observes that it is ethically untenable to expect doctors to face this tradeoff during each patient encounter. He predicts that solutions that recognize cost- effective care as acceptable will be politically and ethically sustainable only if patients as citizens of the larger population accept the need for rationing of limited resources in health care.

John Graham has argued that if the public were actually informed about existing misallocations in resources, they would be startled by the magnitude of discrepancies that exist (Graham, 1996). Ubel (2000) has called for an explicit debate by a broad audience over the moral questions raised by priority-setting and CEA in all their "full and troubling complexity." The idea is that this would force people to recognize value judgments and highlight current policies that create inequitable access.

Daniels and Sabin (2002) call for greater public deliberation and democratic oversight of rationing decisions and the grounds for making them. "Publicity," they argue, is a necessary condition for public acceptance of limit-setting, provided it is done fairly and legitimately. They note that little effort has actually been made to see what transparency produces, and surmise that trust would go *up*, not down, were such a condition to exist. Furthermore, they argue that the tendency to mask the rationale underlying decisions has, in fact, not worked for anyone, that instead it has produced widespread suspicion and the backlash against managed care, and has generally undercut any public sense of fairness. They also dispute the notion that America is different from other countries because it lacks concern about solidarity or sharing, calling this an untested hypothesis and possibly a self-fulfilling prophesy.

Sweeping changes in attitudes may yet occur. The United States may witness a broad shift in the way policy makers think about priority-setting. Practicing physicians may begin to embrace CEA openly as a tool of bedside rationing. Payers may begin appealing more directly to evidence from CEAs when writing contracts or making coverage decisions. The public may become more accepting of the technique, especially if alternative approaches to rationing—such as bureaucratic obstacles and long queues— are seen as even more abhorrent (Weinstein, 2001).

These scenarios seem unlikely, however. Troubled youths are more likely to become troubled adults, or at least unsettled ones. If anything, recent history points to a backlash against the imposition of limits. The public's appetite for managed care has long been eroding (Robinson, 2001). Most recent movements seem headed in the opposite direction, refraining from intruding into the physician–patient relationship, easing restrictions on care, offering broader provider networks, and making it easier for patients to gain access to specialists (Center for Studying Health System Change, 2003). Instead of explicit limits, insurers and employers are opting to put the consumer in charge, armed with information and financial incentives for using health-care resources more prudently (Iglehart, 2002; Galvin and Milstein, 2002). Unlike our neighbors to the north or across the ocean, the United States seems destined to keep CEA at bay, defying the foreign trend like we have resisted the metric system (or universal health care).

Other countries have created national commissions to publicly discuss choices, priorities, and limits in health care. Nothing like this has ever existed in the United States. Where debate does emerge, it tends to focus, not on the public acknowledgment of the problem, but only on inefficiencies and potential market solutions (Daniels and Sabin, 2002). Debates often devolve into rants about "bad governments" or "greedy managed care," rather than honest discussions about the necessity of rationing (Ubel, 2000). The one real exception to the rule occurred in Oregon. And even the Oregon plan, which was greeted much more warmly by Europeans than by Americans, only focused on the state's poorest residents.

The more probable future in the United States is one in which cost-effectiveness information is produced in abundance but seldom used in an explicit way to approve or deny services. Instead, employers and health insurers will probably continue to impose limits in other ways. Society will ration health care not through explicit cost-effectiveness analysis but by increasing cost-sharing arrangements for patients and by rationing quietly, behind the scenes, as harried doctors, nurses, and administrators keep resource constraints in mind when they make everyday decisions, and even nudge families to allow very ill patients to forego intensive medical care and die (Anand, 2003).

Proponents of CEA will continue to push quantification to its limits. They will lament choices made with our hearts, not our heads, and regret that we fall prey to the squeakiest wheel, to public prejudice, media distortions and legal and political concerns (Sheingold, 1998; Paltiel, 2000). One economist recently observed that "there is apparently a great deal of resistance . . . from people who seem to believe that the very process of counting and measuring drains the milk of human kindness out of health care" (Williams, 2001).

But visions of openly prioritizing services based on cost-effectiveness utility ratios are not likely to materialize, at least in the short term. There exists little leadership or political will for it in United States. There is no easy roadmap for change. Simply pressing the point and calling for more rationality won't suffice. Rather, the struggle needs to account for the nature of the resistance and the cultural and institutional obstacles in the peculiar American landscape.

Advancing the debate

Taking the long view. In advancing the debate, one should first take the long view. The need to acknowledge resource constraints is a recent phenomenon that societies have only just begun to address. Daniels and Sabin (2002) point out that public acceptance of limits took place in Sweden, Canada, New Zealand, and other countries only after two or three generations of national health insurance, which created a widespread understanding about the need to share limited resources under politically negotiated budget constraints.

Akehurst (2001) points out that in the United Kingdom, the adoption of CEA occurred only after a significant investment by a "large and vociferous" group of health economists who pushed the paradigm, formed a reservoir of manpower, and generated an "evaluative culture." There was a protracted effort to educate managers within the NHS, and the eventual creation of NICE was preceded by regional Development Evaluation Committees. The movement towards evidence-based medicine accustomed clinicians to careful assessment of the evidence underpinning their actions.

By these lights, the United States may simply be in its early stages of a social learning curve. How to gain a foothold and move forward? The existing rhetoric has generally lacked specific calls for action.

Educating health professionals and the public. One place to start is with education. Physicians are not currently trained about the need to ration or how to ration. They need to be taught that CEA is a technique for increasing value, not simply a mathematical tool wielded by "cold-hearted economists" (Eddy,1992b). Surveys of physicians indicate confusion about how to apply principles of cost-effectiveness analysis, as well as a need to develop consensus on process (Ginsberg et al., 2000; Hershey, 2003).

Formal training about cost-effectiveness analysis in medical and other health professional schools, as well as expansions of fellowships, master's, and doctoral programs are warranted. Eddy (1992d) likens the situation to the medical community's gradual but universal acceptance of statistical techniques, despite the fact that most physicians did not—and do not—comprehend the theory underlying them. The evolution of evidence-based medicine by professional societies offers another possible parallel (Garber, 2001). Having incorporated these principles into the curriculum and culture, the medical establishment would be well served by integrating concepts of decision analysis and cost-effectiveness analysis.

The educational efforts should also extend to regulators, legislators, and the public (Sacramento Health Care, 2001). The various European commissions established to discuss priority-setting in health care offer lessons and some reason for optimism. For one thing, as Daniels and Sabin (2002) note, all encountered controversy initially. Beyond that they provided a roadmap and a demonstrated process and the possibilities for public learning.

Educating the public presents the biggest challenge and the biggest opportunity. Weinstein (2001) argues that an informed population aware of limits is the essential ingredient; that in the end, patients must be at peace with the principle of living within our means.

Finally, even without formal public commissions, there may be institutional policies that could help foster a culture of openness about limit-setting. Daniels and Sabin (2002) point to numerous examples in which private institutions have sought to educate members and to provide a transparent process. Among the examples the authors provide are: Harvard Pilgrim Health Care in Massachusetts, which puts its organizational ethics program meetings on the Web; Allina Health System in Minnesota, which has published an extended statement of principles; Group Health Cooperative in Washington State, which has held public meetings on rationing issues; and Blue Cross Blue Shield of Tennessee, which has published rationales for its policies on its websites.

All of this leaves us with a paradox. How to ration resources honestly in a political environment that doesn't allow policy makers to openly restrict services with evidence of positive health benefit? The Medicare experience suggests that America desperately needs an open debate at a time in which political forces will not allow it. What emerges is CEA's version of the Heisenberg principle: the more transparent and precise we make our rationing process, the harder it is to implement. Simply telling the public that society already rations is insufficient, like an American abroad repeating words in English louder and more slowly to someone who doesn't understand the language. Simply convincing physicians that they already ration (e.g., by not giving the expensive but only marginally better drug as first-line therapy) is also insufficient. We need to find ways to prioritize health services while preserving physicians' and the public's sense of fairness and accounting for political realities.

Physicians and managers understand that resources are limited but they are not willing to acknowledge that they ration. Research shows that physicians, when presented with various clinical vignettes, prefer those reflecting cost-consciousness, even while unwilling to agree that they represent rationing. While insisting that they don't ration, they appeal to "standards of care," even though those are influenced by costs. One physician survey respondent noted that prescribing a low-cost drug as first-line therapy was "not rationing but "delivering sufficient care in a cost-effective manner" (Ubel, 2000, pp. 126–8, 131, 135). Similarly, managed-care plans deny that they ration care but admit that their budgets are constrained (Prosser et al., 2001). A pharmacist defending a new hospital policy of restricting coverage for the expensive sepsis drug Xigris recently said: "Today cost is part of the equation. It's not so much rationing drugs, but using them rationally" (Regalado, 2003). All of this suggests a covert life of cost-effectiveness, one in which the term "cost-effectiveness" cannot easily be used. But this doesn't mean that progress cannot be made.

10

Advice for CEA Practitioners

. . . .

All models are wrong, but some are useful.

—George Box, 1978

To some extent, the problems confronting CEA are methodological. Users need reassurance, not only that analyses are conceptually consistent, but also that the measurement techniques underlying them are valid (Gold et al., 1996). Though a full treatment of methodological advances is beyond the scope of this book, some important areas are highlighted here. Readers interested in exploring the topic in greater detail should consult other references on the subject (e.g., Drummond and McGuire, 2001).

Technical Improvements

Methods for estimating costs

One way to enhance the acceptability of CEAs is to improve the quality of the data inputs. As detailed in chapter 4, the methods that analysts have employed for estimating costs in existing CEAs have varied over the years. Analysts have differed considerably in the ways that they have conceptualized and estimated costs. Many studies have lacked transparency in their approaches.

Standardization in the costing methods used and how they are reported would clearly help. So, too, would paying more attention to practical issues confronting decision makers. Many CEAs have failed to consider the cost of implementing the services in question, or have neglected other factors that may alter cost-effectiveness, such as the availability of an intervention, the mix and quality of inputs, local prices, and the supporting institutional framework (Murray et al., 2000). More attention to these factors is needed so that policy makers can identify the full resource implications of implementing interventions that are shown to be cost-effective, and the costs of steps needed to add, modify, or eliminate services (Hutubessy et al., 2002).

CEAs alongside randomized controlled trials

An area of growing interest involves collecting economic and health outcomes information alongside clinical information in randomized controlled trials (RCTs) (Drummond and Stoddart, 1984; Adams et al., 1992; Pritchard, 1999). These studies follow the accepted traditions of clinical trials, with rigorous scientific design, pre-specified endpoints, and even formal testing of hypotheses. As a consequence they should help increase the faith that decision makers place in CEAs (Ramsey et al., 2001).

Conducting CEAs alongside RCTs also raises challenges. For one thing, they can be expensive and potentially burdensome to patients. Sample size requirements are typically greater for economic trials than for purely clinical studies, because there is more variation around economic endpoints measured, such as hospitalization, than around clinical endpoints. The purposes of clinical trials and CEAs are often distinct and occasionally in conflict: where clinical trials are usually conducted to test new drugs against a placebo to meet FDA requirements that drugs be safe and effective, CEAs are undertaken to compare new treatments with the best existing alternative and to guide decisions by reimbursement authorities (Ramsey et al., 2001; Tunis et al., 2003). As a result, simply adding economic variables to existing randomized clinical trial may not yield helpful results.

Another concern is that care provided in clinical trials may not represent typical medical practice because patients selected for trials are atypical (e.g., they may be healthier than other patients with the disease under investigation), because care is not typical (because clinicians involved in trials tend to be experts in their field and thus not representative of average practice patterns), or because greater scrutiny of patients in a trial setting could result in a higher-than-average probability of detecting disease (Ramsey et al., 2001). Thus, decision makers rely upon models even in situations where "hard" evidence, such as results from randomized controlled trials, is available.

Models in cost-effectiveness analyses

Decisions must always be made in the face of uncertainty. Frequently, policy makers don't have the luxury of waiting for data from randomized controlled trials. The costs associated with waiting can be substantial in terms of potential foregone benefits. Thus, policy makers often turn to models to inform their choices. The alternative of waiting for direct evidence can result in years of missed opportunity to save lives and improve health. The alternative of relying on expert judgment without models risks errors due to the known limitations of human judgment in choices that involve complex combinations of probabilities and consequences (Tversky and Kahneman, 1981; Sandberg et al., 2003).

Models are ubiquitous in CEAs. CEAs rely on models to extrapolate from surrogate markers used in clinical trials (e.g., acute coronary events, cancer progression, or HIV-RNA rebound) to long-term endpoints, such as life expectancy and total economic costs. Even when clinical trials contain survival as a primary endpoint, decision makers employ models—implicitly if not explicitly—to project results to future events and to population subgroups excluded from the trial. Decision makers also find models helpful for projecting "what if" scenarios and in exploring the degree of uncertainty surrounding study parameters (Sandberg et al., 2003).

A key area for further research is to improve the internal validity of models, to better calibrate them (to ensure that inputs and outputs are consistent with available data), and to validate them (by comparing predictions of models with actual data collected after the fact) (Weinstein et al., 2001b; Thompson et al., 2002).

Characterizing and presenting uncertainty in CEAs

The advent of economic analyses of information collected alongside clinical trials—and the availability of patient-level data on both costs and effects—has led to advances in the use of statistical methods, including sample size and power estimation (see, for example, O'Brien et al., 1994; Willan and O'Brien, 1996; Polsky et al., 1997; Briggs, 1997; Briggs et al., 2002).

On the cost side, researchers have worked on statistical models to explain cost distributions and have improved methods to handle missing data while adjusting for co-variates and predicting costs in the followup period of the trial. They have also developed approaches to account for protocol-induced costs (extra costs such as testing and monitoring that are precipitated by the trial itself) (Etzioni et al., 1999; Ramsey et al., 2001; Briggs et al., 2002).

One of the most active areas of research has involved methods to analyze and present uncertainty in cost-effectiveness analyses (Claxton and Posnett, 1996; Claxton, 1999; Briggs et al., 2002). Investigators have established methods of calculating confidence intervals for cost-effectiveness ratios when patient-level data on costs and effects are available to generate empirical distributions of cost-effectiveness.

Improving the analysis and characterization of uncertainty is one of the most important areas for the field. Some researchers have proposed using "net benefit statistics" as a framework for handling uncertainty in CEA (Stinnett and Mullahy, 1998). The net health benefit (NHB) presents a rearrangement of the cost-effectiveness ratio to turn it into a simple linear expression:

$$\text{NHB} = (E_1 - E_0) - (C_1 - C_0)/\lambda$$

where E_1 and C_1 represent the effectiveness and cost of intervention 1; E_0 and C_0 represent the effectiveness and cost of intervention 0; and λ represents societal willingness to pay for health gains (e.g., QALYs).

Net benefit avoids certain calculation problems with ratio-based statistics. For example, incremental C/E ratios as commonly calculated, can be negative (e.g., –$20,000/QALY), which is problematic because it says nothing about whether the negative sign is attributed to the numerator or denominator of the ratio. In contrast the NHB turns the ratio into a simple decision rule: if NHB > 0, the new program or technology should be adopted. Net benefit has other purported advantages: it makes the statistic more tractable and its sample distribution much better behaved, and it simplifies sample size calculations (Briggs et al., 2002). Its developers have argued that a key advantage is that it forces an explicit consideration of λ (Stinnett and Mullahy, 1998).

In fact, though, we know little about how decision makers process cost-effectiveness information, including information about net health benefits. The net benefit approach may be problematic for policy makers precisely because it forces an explicit consideration of societal willingness to pay. American policy makers may be unwilling to accept a public declaration of a rigid cost-effectiveness threshold such as $50,000/QALY. More exploration of the matter is needed.

Related to the net benefit framework is the idea of *acceptability curves*, which provide a way of summarizing evidence that supports the cost-effectiveness of a particular intervention as a function of a decision maker's willingness to pay for the benefits produced (Fig. 10–1) (Briggs et al., 2002). The idea is that, unlike other displays of cost-effectiveness information, acceptability curves directly address the question at hand for policy makers: How likely is it that the new intervention is cost-effective? Acceptability

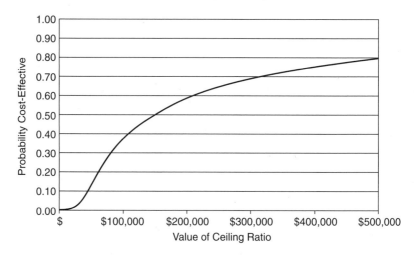

Figure 10–1.   Cost-effectiveness acceptability curve.

curves may thus offer an important innovation in the presentation of infor-mation about uncertainty. However, more research is needed into how they are viewed and used by policy makers.

Valuing health outcomes

Improving the measurement of health values has been an extremely active area of research. Researchers have worked actively for years to develop better methods for eliciting preference weights for use in the calculation of QALYs.[1] Considerable research has tested the validity and reliability of the various techniques for measuring health and the feasibility of eliciting responses (Torrance, 1982; Torrance, 1986; Gold et al., 1996).

Researchers have excelled in developing and eliciting preferences for various states of health. To a large extent, though, they have not followed through in exploring whether the use of these elicited preferences in CEAs reflect how people want to allocate health resources.

As noted in chapter 1, researchers have used a number of techniques over the years to construct these quality weights, including the "standard gamble" or "time tradeoff" techniques, which involve asking respondents to value health states by considering explicitly how much they would be willing to sacrifice to avoid being in a particular health state. An alternative technique is the rating scale in which respondents are asked to express the strength of their preferences for particular health states by marking a point on a scale.

In comparison to the standard gamble, the time tradeoff technique has proved to be relatively valid, while the rating scale has not (Torrance, 1976). In general, rating scales, while easy to use, are subject to measurement bias (Torrance et al., 1996). A number of studies have shown that different elicitation methods lead to different preference weights. Most indicate that standard gamble scores are greater than time tradeoff scores, which are in turn greater than scores from rating scales (Bleichrodt and Johannesson, 1997; Drummond et al., 1997, Hornberger et al., 1992; Nease et al., 1995; O'Leary et al., 1995; Van Wijck et al., 1998). Numerous researchers have explored how the precise method of elicitation influences results.[2]

Research groups continue to refine universal or "generic" health-state classification systems, such as the Health Utilities Index (HUI) (Torrance et al., 1996; Feeny et al., 2002), the Quality of Well-Being Scale (Kaplan et al., 1989), and the EuroQol (EQ5D) (EuroQol Group, 1990). These systems are designed to be complete and general enough to apply across many different types of conditions and treatments. They provide an indirect means of obtaining preference weights: patients are assigned a health state classification based on responses to health status questionnaires, and pre-specified preference weights obtained from other populations are then applied.

But the systems differ in terms of how they define the relevant domains or attributes of health, as well as the techniques used for obtaining preference weights. For example, the Health Utilities Index contains eight attributes—vision, hearing, speech, ambulation, dexterity, emotion, cognition, and pain—with five to six levels of functioning per attribute. Preference measurements are based on the visual analog scale and the standard gamble instruments, and were collected from a population sample in Hamilton, Ontario. The EQ5D contains five attributes—mobility, self-care, main activity, usual activity, pain/discomfort, and anxiety/depression—with three levels per attribute. The scoring function for preferences is based on the time tradeoff technique on a random sample of the adult population in the United Kingdom. Studies have revealed both similarities and differences in preference weights obtained by using different instruments in the same population (Glick et al., 1999; Nord, 1996), and in preferences obtained with generic instruments versus preferences assessed directly (Bosch et al., 1994; Bosch et al., 1996; Gabriel et al., 1999, Tsevat, 1996).

A great deal of work has been conducted to examine and compare patients' preferences to preferences of non-patients. Patients afflicted with a specific condition tend to place a higher value on their own health states compared to the values non-patients place when evaluating the the condition (Sackett, 1978; Epstein et al., 1989; Gabriel et al., 1999), though similarities in preferences have also been reported between patients and non-patients (Balaban, 1986; Llewellyn-Thomas, 1984; Patrick, 1985; Revicki, 1996). The general explanation for disparities between patients and non-patients is that patients adapt in order to accommodate their limitations and alter their goals and expectations (Gold et al., 1996). Researchers have also reported that patient values are higher than their surrogates believe (Tsevat, 1995; Tsevat, 1996). Wide individual-to-individual variations in health values, however, are common (Fryback, 1993; Nease et al., 1995; Tsevat et al., 1998).

Researchers have studied a number of options for deriving information on patients' preferences from clinical trials, including the use of direct utility assessments (Bombadier et al., 1986; Laupacis, 1991), as well as generic health-state classification systems (Feeny et al., 1989). The relationship between psychometric health-status measures (e.g., the Short Form (SF)-36) and preference measures has also been explored (Brazier et al., 1993; Gondek et al., 1998). Several researchers have developed a set of health-related quality-of-life scores for chronic conditions based on nationally representative U.S. data from the National Health Interview Survey (Gold et al., 1998). Elsewhere, researchers have developed a comprehensive catalogue of preference weights using secondary data from published cost-utility analyses (Bell et al., 2001).

While researchers have focused attention on measuring individual preferences for health states for use in QALY estimates, however, they have paid much less attention to whether QALYs adequately reflect public preferences for rationing. Nord (1999) argues that QALYs haven't really grown up since they were first proposed in the early Seventies, when there was no empirical evidence or strong inquiry into their theoretical foundations. Economists who proposed QALYs, like the Panel on Cost-Effectiveness, which recommended them, have focused on efficiency concerns and paid little attention to issues of fairness and other problems they raise.

More attention to the matter is warranted to explore community values for priority-setting and to adapt QALY measurement for CEA. Research shows, for example, that people want to give priority to severely ill patients, or avoid discrimination against people with limited treatment potential due to disabilities (Ubel, 2000).

Many have called for cost-effectiveness analysis to formally consider values other than efficiency, such as fairness or equity (e.g., Dolan, 1998; Nord, 1999; Federal Budget Submission, 2002). Analysts, for example, could weight QALYs gained by particular subgroups to incorporate equity considerations, or they could weight changes in QALYs more heavily for members whose initial level of health is lower (Ubel, 2000). Utilities could be rescaled, for example, to give more weight to the severely ill, that is, a change in utility from 0.1 to 0.2 could be given more weight than a change, say, from 0.7 to 0.8. Williams (1997) has proposed equity weights for QALYs that account for people's age in order to address what he terms a "fair innings" concern that everyone is entitled to a "normal" span of life.

Utility estimates could accommodate concerns about distributive effects by aggregating individual utilities in ways other than a simple sum of QALYs; for example, by maximizing the utility of the worst-off individuals (the maximin rule) (Gold et al., 1996, p. 35). Analysts could even calculate equity separately and display equity estimates alongside utilities, so that decision makers would consider both numbers (Ubel, 2000, p. 172). At the very least, qualitative descriptions of equity and fairness might be presented to decision makers.[3]

Other approaches are also possible. One alternative is the measurement of "person tradeoffs" as a way of enabling analysts to value a broader range of outcomes (Nord, 1999). Under the approach, community samples are asked to express the number of people obtaining one kind of health outcome that would be considered equivalent to a given number of people obtaining another outcome. The technique may allow more natural consideration of tradeoffs involved for moderate or slight improvements in health than is possible with individual utility approaches, though it clearly raises challenges as well. Other alternatives to QALYs include healthy-years equivalents (HYEs) (Mehrez and Gafni, 1989), saved young life equivalents (SAVEs) (Nord, 1992), and disability-adjusted life years (DALYs) (Murray, 1994), though it is important to note that each of the options has its own limitations and is subject to debate (Gold et al., 1996).[4]

The limits of technical adjustments

Advances in CEA methodology and presentation promise more precise measurement techniques. The innovations will undoubtedly help the field gain a reputation for more rigor and thoughtfulness.

Even with technical improvements, though, CEAs will always face challenges because the exercise involves value considerations—not simply whether service A is more effective than B, but whether A is worth the investment.

Alternative approaches to cost-utility analyses all carry their own problems, imposing their own set of value judgments. For all the criticism of QALYs, no acceptable alternative has arisen. There has been little movement in the field to adopt equity weightings, for example, or any other proposed innovation.

The *Panel on Cost-Effectiveness* recommended that analysts use an overarching "rule of reason": a "reasonableness" standard in conducting CEAs. For example, analysts should be reasonable in determining how far to estimate the outward ripples of an intervention's costs and effects. The rule of reason offers an eminently sensible suggestion, but it is often too vague to provide meaningful guidance.

Even with the best methodical improvements and the most reasonable assumptions, the field needs more consideration of the institutions and infrastructure surrounding the use of CEA. What matters more than technical improvements are the policies under which decision makers consider putting CEAs to use.

When Bad Things Happen to Good Methodology

"We are stuck with cost-effectiveness analyses and trying to make them honest," two leading critics of the field recently grumbled (Rennie and Luft, 2000). Everyone seems to agree that concerns about the comparability and credibility of cost-effectiveness analyses will persist without further improvements in the field. The lack of clarity makes it difficult for readers to understand study objectives and to judge the quality and appropriateness of results (Siegel et al., 1996). Poor reporting practices, even more than unresolved technical issues, may explain lingering suspicions about cost-utility analyses and what some have termed the "lack of respect" for the field (Reinhardt, 1997). They may also be easier to fix than the resolution of controversial theoretical or technical questions about estimation methods.

Experience suggests, however, that changing practice will not be easy. Conventional peer review has not tended to ease CEA's credibility problem. Numerous studies document that published CEAs have not adhered to recommended protocols and that the problem has persisted over time (Udvarhelyi et al., 1992; Neumann et al., 1997; Jefferson et al., 1998; Gerard et al., 1999; Gerard, 1992; Brown and Fintor, 1993; Nord, 1993a; Mason, 1994; Adams et al., 1992; Briggs and Sculpher, 1995; Blackmore and Magid, 1997; Balas, 1998). Neumann et al. (2000a), for example, found that between 1976 and 1997, over one third of published cost-utility analyses did not disclose their sources of funding. Almost half did not clearly state the study perspective. Only 46.1% correctly reported incremental cost-effectiveness ratios. In general, they found considerable variation in the way that costs and preference weights have been reported.

Analysts usually have not complied with established standards for reporting CEAs, and journal editors have not enforced them. Protocols to ensure the rigor and transparency of published CEAs have existed for many years. Independent task forces have called for the full disclosure of all commercial ties and funding support and whether any restrictions were placed on authors, such as control of and access to data, publication rights, and sponsors' right to review (Task Force on Principles for Economic Analyses, 1995). Leading medical journals have published guidelines calling for transparency in reporting study methods, as well as protocols for releasing model software and data for peer review, and making technical reports available (Siegel et al., 1996). Checklists for reviewers and journal editors have been published. However, they often fail to adhere to their own guidelines (Jefferson et al., 1998).

It is not at all clear that traditional peer review is up to the task. Even with access to all the data and models, it took Australian pharmaceutical reimbursement authorities two weeks to thoroughly review cost-effectiveness analyses, for example (Hill et al., 2000), much more time than any reasonable peer reviewer would spend.

One option for change involves the *New England Journal of Medicine*'s strategy of banning authors of CEAs with a direct financial stake in study results (Kassirer and Angell, 1994). But this approach amounts to a declaration of defeat and a peculiar form of discrimination (industry profiling?). Journal editors should decide whether cost-effectiveness analysis is a legitimate field of scientific inquiry or not. They should not selectively exclude authors on the basis of their professional backgrounds.

Instead, leaders in the field should renew calls to improve the quality of published analyses, and also articulate clear objectives for the field and a timetable for meeting them. For example, they might agree that all published CEAs by 2010 should clearly delineate the study perspective, the methods used to estimate costs and health benefits, and the source of funding. All abstracts of CEAs should clearly state the intervention under investigation, as well as the comparator, target population, and study perspective (Rosen et al., 2003). Researchers should regularly monitor the field to determine progress towards the goals. Journals, grant-making organizations, and government agencies should publicly adopt and enforce the policies.

Scoring systems to evaluate the quality of health economic analyses may help discriminate higher- from lower-quality studies and be useful to journal editors, as well as decision makers themselves (e.g., Fang et al., 2003). More work on their validation and application is required, however (Ofman et al., 2003; Motheral, 2003).

There is some evidence that published cost-effectiveness analyses are improving. Neumann et al. (2000a) reported steady improvement in a number of measures, including clearly stating the study perspective, providing a diagram of the event pathway, and discussing study limitations. More recent data confirm the trends (Fig. 10–2).

Evidence also suggests that the quality of CEAs improves with the experience of the journal publishing them. Neumann et al. (2000a) also found that a journal's experience with CEA was a good predictor of the overall quality of its reporting practices.[5] The publication of cost-utility analyses in "low-volume" journals (journals that have published three or fewer cost-utility analyses) has continued in recent years, which may explain why the percentage of articles using good reporting practices has not improved more over time.

The success of initiatives to improve the methods and reporting of randomized trials and systematic reviews may offer models for CEAs (Rennie and Luft, 2000; Jefferson and Demicheli, 2002). Rennie and Luft (2000) point out that efforts to provide a formal systematic structure in order to reduce selection bias and make studies more transparent revolutionized the reporting of meta-analyses and other systematic reviews.

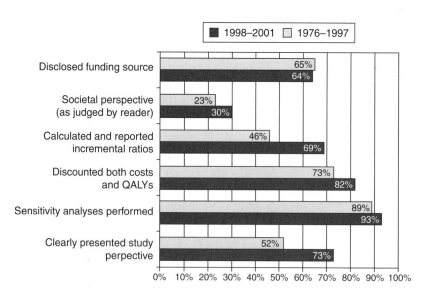

Figure 10–2. Improvements in CUAs over time. *Source*: CEA Registry, 2003 (www.hsph.harvard.edu/cearegistry).

Beyond that, editors could insist that authors provide details about the CEA on the journal's website themselves so that their assumptions and data can be reviewed, as in the discovery process in lawsuits, whereby each side has access to the underlying data that may be presented (Rennie and Luft, 2000; Lyles, 2001). Concerns about confidentiality and intellectual property raise challenges, but this is an area worth exploring.

Improving the Translation of CEAs

Relatively little attention has been paid to the translation of CEA results, even though it is clear that decision makers have infrequently used the information and that physicians are often confused by cost-effectiveness ratios (e.g., Hershey et al., 2003).

A key area for exploration involves the presentation of uncertainty. As noted above, analysts have proposed using the cost-effectiveness plane as a device to present and explore the implications of uncertainty, to give the clearest intuitive understanding of the implications of uncertainty for the analysis (Briggs et al., 2002). Investigators have proposed using acceptability curves, which show the weight of evidence for the intervention being cost-effective for all possible values of the cost-effectiveness threshold (the willingness to pay for life years or QALYs) (Briggs, 2002). In other words, how likely is it that the intervention is cost-effective? League tables generally do not display any information about uncertainty. In the future, analysts might present confidence limits for cost-effectiveness ratios, displaying both the mean and variance of the incremental cost-effectiveness ratios, so that a risk-averse decision maker can trade off the expected value with the risk of not achieving that value (Mauskopf et al., 2003).

Mauskopf et al. (2003) have recommended other changes in league tables, such as presenting estimates of the magnitude of incremental costs and benefits per patient as well as the overall incremental cost-effectiveness ratios, and presenting cost-effectiveness ratios for different population subgroups if the cost-effectiveness varies by subgroup. They also suggest that analysts present annual budget impact estimates for the new treatment for the total population as well as the cost-effectiveness ratio for a representative individual.

Understanding perceptions of cost-effectiveness

Several themes emerge from the study of risk perception that may hold lessons for the translation of cost-effectiveness analysis. In developing risk perceptions, people pay attention to the social and subjective nature of risk, not just the quantitative estimates involved (Slovic, 1987). Paul Slovic (1987, 1989) has observed that the public views risk in a broader context than scientific fact, mixing value judgments, pre-formed preferences, and personal anecdotes with intellectual understanding and acceptance of the facts, often in ways that are not easy to predict.

Another theme is that the public systematically over- or underestimates certain risks. People seem to worry about the "wrong" risks, often expressing greater concern about risks of smaller magnitude, such as environmental contaminants, chemical toxicity, rare infectious diseases, or additives in food, than about risks of greater magnitude, such as smoking or alcohol abuse (Graham and Weiner, 1996; Samsa et al., 1997; Ayanian and Cleary, 1999). This reflects emotional factors such as dread or one's sense of voluntariness or controllability, which play a large role in the perception of risk (Slovic, 1987).

In general, *affect* comes before explicit judgments of risks and benefits are made (Finucane et al., 2000). Investigators have also found gender differences in risk perception: women are more concerned about adverse consequences and men more tolerant of risk (Graham and Wiener, 1996). A third theme is that misperceptions of risk are aggravated by the use of jargon and abstraction and there is a general lack of clarity in the presentation of information.

The same themes may apply to CEA. In developing their intuitions about cost-effectiveness, people may focus on social factors, personal anecdotes, and pre-formed preferences. These may lead them to believe, incorrectly, that certain services are more cost-effective than others, or to dismiss cost-effectiveness in favor of other considerations. Differences in intuitions about cost-effectiveness, or about the uncertainty surrounding estimates of cost-effectiveness, may relate to gender, age, or profession.

These differences may persist across diseases or types of interventions. Experiences in the United Kingdom and Australia suggest that decision makers do not hold to fixed, absolute cost-effectiveness thresholds. Instead, they exercise discretion and make allowances for special cases. Varied factors may influence them, including the degree of uncertainty about results, the availability of alternative treatments, the larger community's preferences, and the seriousness of the disease or condition in question (George et al., 2001). George et al. (2001) note that a wider range of objectives than simply maximizing health gain at minimum cost is at work, one where factors such as equity, whether a treatment is for a life-threatening condition, access, and affordability considerations and financial implications for government influence decisions.

But how important is each factor and when do they come into play? In some cases, physicians may not prescribe certain medications because they do not believe them to be cost-effective. In others they may prescribe them despite the fact that they are not cost-effective. This may have been the case in NICE's decision on Alzheimer's drugs, which seems to reflect a preference for giving patients some access to the medications despite equivocal data on cost-effectiveness. Given the difficulties of predicting in advance who will respond to treatment, physicians may deem it important to give all patients a chance and then selectively withdraw the drug from those who do not respond.

Communicating cost-effectiveness information

The field of risk communication may also offer important lessons. Healthcare professionals face a constant challenge in translating data about risks and probabilities into the language of patients (Herrier, 1995; Bottorff et al., 1998, Bogardus et al., 1999; Schwartz et al., 1997). Researchers have found that words and pictures are important in explaining risks (Nakao, 1983; Bogardus et al., 1999; Woloshin et al., 2000). The context and the way a risk is described shapes patients' perceptions (Gurm et al., 2000).

Researchers have long known that the framing of risks influences perceptions (Tversky and Kahneman, 1981; McNeil et al., 1982). They have found that physicians see therapy as more effective when shown *relative* risk data and less effective when shown *absolute* risk of an outcome (Naylor et al., 1992). Morris and Hammitt (2001) recently reported that people seem willing to pay more for a longevity benefit expressed as a life expectancy gain than as a continuing reduction in annual mortality risk.

Communicating risks about cancer can present special challenges (Fischhoff, 1999; Fong et al., 1999). Breast cancer is a feared disease in women, and its risk is often overestimated (Vogel, 1999). Schwartz et al. (1997) found that few women could accurately apply risk information from mammography when it was presented as absolute risk.

How to translate and communicate cost-effectiveness information needs more serious inquiry along these lines. Despite efforts to promote the concept of cost-effectiveness, we know very little about how decision makers process the information. It is cognitively difficult for decision makers to develop an intuitive feeling for what constitutes a large or small life-expectancy gain (Wright and Weinstein, 1998) and thus to have accurate intuitions about cost-effectiveness. We need to better understand how framing affects cost-effectiveness perceptions and how to develop ways to better communicate the data.

Repackaging the term

The field could also benefit from more fundamental changes in how it presents itself. Some have argued, on theoretical grounds, for the adoption of cost-benefit analysis (CBA) rather than cost-effectiveness analysis (Pauly, 1995). In CBA, analysts estimate the net social benefit of a program or intervention as the incremental benefit of a program minus the incremental cost. All costs and benefits are measured in monetary units (e.g., dollars). Health benefits can be valued, according to economic principles, by estimating how much individuals are willing to pay for them. Conceivably, this approach offers a more politically acceptable alternative to CEA because it leads to a simple decision rule: if a program's net benefits exceed its net costs, then it should be adopted.

As noted in chapter 2, CBA raises measurement difficulties and ethical dilemmas, however, because it requires the monetary valuation of health benefits. Notably, the charge given to the Panel on Cost-Effectiveness by the U.S. Public Health Service was to examine cost-effectiveness analysis and not cost-benefit analysis (Weinstein, personal communication, February 2003). Moreover, the number of published CEAs has vastly outpaced the number of CBAs over time (see Figure 2–1).

The "net-health benefit" approach, in which analysts select a willingness to pay for a quality-adjusted life year (QALY) and present data in a format similar to that of CBA, has been advanced as a more acceptable alternative (Stinnett and Mullahy, 1998). The explicit declaration of the societal cost-effectiveness threshold is touted as one of the benefits of the approach because it forces decision makers to confront the issue of opportunity costs. More likely, though, it is an impediment because the explicit valuation exercise is precisely what decision makers seek to avoid. Moreover, there is no agreement on which threshold to use (Winkelmeyer and Neumann, 2002). To date, relatively few net-health benefit analyses have been published.

Another alternative involves changing, not the approach itself, but the way the cost-effectiveness ratio is presented. For example, analysts might invert the ratio and present the number of QALYs obtained per dollar invested, rather than costs per QALY achieved. The idea is not new (Eddy, 1992a). Decision makers might find the "E/C ratio" attractive because it presents the approach as a tool for improving health within a budget, rather than as a cost-cutting technique. On the downside, the term is unfamiliar. Eddy (1992a) long ago pointed out that "it's easiest to bow to the common usage and refer to the cost-effectiveness ratio."

More important, the E/C ratio doesn't address what might be a more fundamental concern: ridding the term of the word *cost*. As long as the word *cost* inhabits the phrase, the approach will be perceived as a technique for drawing limits and saving money, rather than enhancing value. David Eddy's conversation with his father captures the problem. Maxon Eddy observes: "The word *cost* is prominent in both cost-effectiveness analysis and cost-benefit analysis. Isn't cost-effectiveness analysis just a smoke-screen for cutting costs at the expense of quality?" (Eddy 1992a).

This suggests that more education and promotion alone will be insufficient; that the way forward will involve thinking creatively about the term *cost-effectiveness*, and perhaps a measure of scientific rebranding to repackage the phrase. While *cost-effectiveness* appeals to the head, analysts also need to appeal to the heart. The debate over getting value in health care needs to be waged in terms of health, not in terms of costs.

Some will object that this is exactly the wrong approach, that the field requires brutal honesty rather than obfuscation and cosmetic change. Asch and Ubel (1997) have argued, "If there is to be a resolution to the debate about compromise in clinical care, it must come from discussion of what actually happens, rather than of the language used to describe it."

Language matters, however, and may matter a lot in this context. If cost-effectiveness were a commercial product, it would have failed by now, at least in the United States. As noted in chapter 3, one health plan that used *cost-effectiveness* in its mission statement removed the offending phrase as too controversial. U.S. policy makers who worry about public opinion and the political arena have already voted with their actions, avoiding the term *cost-effectiveness* in public documents, and resorting to euphemisms. Medicare officials talk about covering "appropriate" care or "truly beneficial services," but never mention the words "cost-effective."

The medical and public health communities have precedents for re-branding terms. NMRs became MRIs to address consumer fears associated with the word "nuclear." The National Highway Traffic Safety Administration reframed the problem of traffic injuries as a public health issue to emphasize that motor vehicle crashes were predictable and preventable (NHTSA, 1999). Marketers devote enormous efforts and resources to understanding how the public reacts to different words and phrases, and to branding products. Over time "used cars" have become "pre-owned," and old Coke became "classic" Coke. The CEA field would benefit from a vigorous debate on the subject.

CEAs might be called something else, perhaps *value analysis*. Another option is *investment-effectiveness analysis*, which implies resources' being used to purchase health rather than to save money (David Ropeik, personal communication, 2001). Medicare officials have used the word "comparability" and "comparative effectiveness" (see Chapter 11).

Private insurers have also gravitated toward the concept of *comparability*, if not yet the term: when covering new drugs, they typically determine therapeutic equivalence first and then begin negotiating, with a competitive bidding process. That is, they consider costs if two services are considered equally effective. If the advance is deemed a clinical breakthrough, they grant a premium price. This approach provides them the veil they need for political acceptability.

Are We Asking the Right Questions?

Are we studying what matters?

A final question concerns whether the field is targeting resources for CEAs efficiently. Research suggests that the CEA field focuses too much attention on medications and surgery rather than on health education or disease-management programs, which could offer greater health gains per research dollar expended (Neumann and Levine, 2002). Existing cost-utility analyses cover a wide range of interventions, though pharmaceuticals (40%) and surgical procedures (16%) account for the majority (Fig. 10–3).

Data suggest that these studies may reflect the narrow interests of individual researchers or funders rather than society's most pressing health

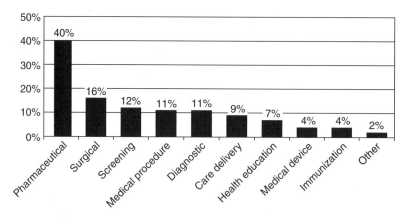

Figure 10–3.   Cost-utility analyses by type of intervention, 1976–2001 (n = 522). *Source*: CEA Registry, 2003 (www.hsph.harvard.edu/cearegistry).

needs. A recent study compared rankings of the most common diseases covered by published CUAs to rankings of disease burden in the United States, measured by underlying cause of death (World Health Organization, 2002) by disability-adjusted life years (DALYs) (World Health Organization, 2002), and by health expenditure (AHRQ, 2003; Cohen, 2003).

Relative to disease burden, the disease areas covered by published CUAs are disproportionately concentrated in certain areas, such as diabetes, breast cancer, and HIV/AIDS, while other areas are underrepresented, such as depression and bipolar disorder, injuries, substance-abuse disorders, chronic obstructive pulmonary disease, Alzheimer's disease and dementias, lung cancer, and asthma (Figs. 10–4, 10–5, 10–6).

Moving from disease burden to goals specified in the U.S. Department of Health and Human Service's Healthy People 2010 report (*Healthy People 2010*), the data suggest that many of the goals for modifiable risk factors have been largely overlooked in the CUA literature. Few CUAs have targeted key *Healthy People 2010* areas such as physical activity, environmental exposures, or tobacco use (Fig. 10–7).

The value of value-of-information analysis

By themselves, discrepancies between diseases addressed by CUAs and diseases of highest burden do not tell a complete story. Disease burden

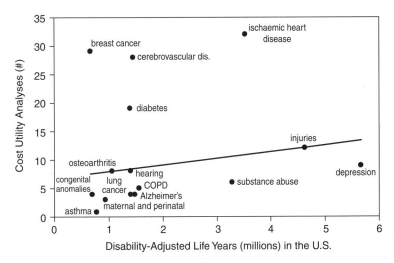

Figure 10–4.   Relationship between diseases' disability-adjusted life years in 2002 and diseases covered by published CUAs. *Source*: CEA Registry, 2003 (www.hsph.harvard.edu/cearegistry).

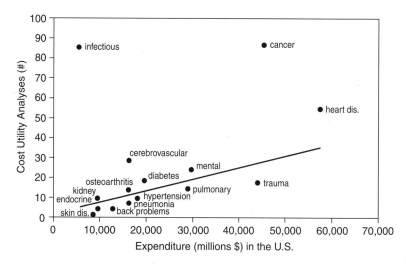

Figure 10–5.   Relationship between expenditure by diagnostic category in the U.S. in 1997 and diseases covered by published CUAs. *Source*: CEA Registry, 2003 (www.hsph.harvard.edu/cearegistry).

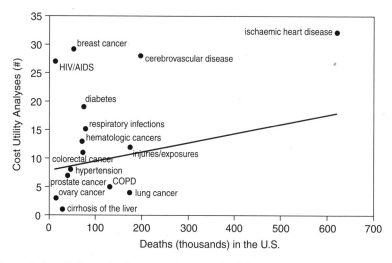

Figure 10–6.   Relationship between causes of death by diagnostic category in 2002 and diseases covered by published CUAs. *Source*: CEA Registry, 2003 (www. hsph.harvard.edu/cearegistry).

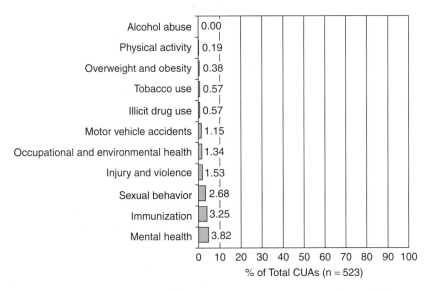

Figure 10–7.   Published CUAs by Healthy People 2010 Priorities. *Source*: CEA Registry, 2003 (www.hsph.harvard.edu/cearegistry).

data say nothing about opportunities for research, for example. It may be possible that there are simply few effective or cost-effective interventions for, say, lung cancer, which explains why few investigators have undertaken CUAs on the topic. It is also possible that interventions in a particular area are well established and known to be cost-effective, so that conducting additional cost-effectiveness research may not be worthwhile. Furthermore, CUA research in certain areas, such as substance abuse disorders, could be inherently more difficult due to the lack of data on effective interventions, or the challenges of obtaining utility weights for abuse-related health states.

The reasons for any society to conduct a cost-effectiveness analysis are to influence decision making to move in the direction of more cost-effective care. In economic terms, the marginal productivity of investments in CUAs should be considered—in other words, whether an additional dollar invested in a CUA of breast cancer treatment is likely to produce more returns than an additional dollar invested in a CUA of a substance-abuse prevention strategy (Hatziandreu et al., 1988).

Decisions about prioritizing investments in research must take many objectives into account. Disease burden is only one of five criteria used in considering NIH funding priorities, for example. The others are scientific opportunity, the scientific quality of research in the area, the probability of success, and the maintenance of a diverse research portfolio (Gross et al., 1999).

Other important societal values may not be captured by aggregated indexes such as disease burden measures. Society's commitment to research may reflect public perceptions and anxiety about certain types of health risk, particularly those that are new, unfamiliar, and potentially catastrophic (Hatziandreu et al., 1988; Slovic, 1987). Investments in CUAs may also reflect concerns about areas of rapid expenditure growth (e.g., pharmaceuticals). Even taking such factors into account, however, the discrepancies raise questions about the priorities reflected in the CUA literature to date.

The predominance of pharmaceutical therapies, which are 40% of the CUA sample yet constitute only 10% of overall health spending (Levitt et al., 2001), is a good example. Cost-effectiveness researchers, often funded by the pharmaceutical industry, have spent a lot of time analyzing whether pharmaceuticals are cost-effective, and relatively less time on other types of interventions. On the other hand, pharmaceuticals could be important in ways that justify their attention. They could be key drivers of health improvements in the major disease areas covered, or key contributors to cost savings if their use offsets more expensive types of care.

It is possible that priorities for CUAs reflect other factors, such as media coverage or the strength of advocacy groups, which may explain the preponderance of research on breast cancer and HIV/AIDs, and the low volume of studies of injuries, diet and physical activity, and motor vehicle injuries. These findings are consistent with other studies that show disparities between government funding for research and diseases with the highest burden (Gross et al,. 1999; Hatziandreu et al., 1988; Michaud et al., 2001).

Various approaches have been offered to set priorities in evaluative research over the years, including methods of explicitly quantifying the gains from research. Phelps and Parente (1990), for example, developed an index of expected gain from research, which incorporates spending levels for a particular condition and the degree of variation in intervention strategies as a way of establishing a first-cut priority-assessment method. Variation is used as a proxy measure for the opportunity for research to eliminate uncertainty associated with a particular technology. Areas with high spending and large variation are thus given higher priority.

Other researchers have attempted to quantify more explicitly the impact of research itself. They have explored methods for quantifying the cost-effectiveness of proposed cost-effectiveness research, by measuring a CEA's impact on a service's use and its ultimate consequences for the population health burden (Claxton, 2001; Weinstein, 1983; Detsky, 1989).

Researchers have proposed a value-of-information framework as a way to determine whether society is spending its resources for evaluative research efficiently (Fenwick et al., 2003). They emphasize that information from research is valuable because it reduces the uncertainty in decisions about health-care policy and practice. Reducing uncertainty through evaluative research is thus valuable because it reduces the expected costs (opportunity losses) associated with health policy decisions. The question of whether to fund additional CUAs in a particular area can be described as judging the cost of the additional research against the gains associated with reducing the uncertainty, and thus the expected costs of making the wrong decision (Fenwick, 2003).

Cost-effectiveness research can also be useful in correcting mismatches between optimal care and actual practice, even if the CEA itself does not reduce uncertainty or involve primary data collection. The process of conducting a CEA may itself generate new information that yields insights. The publication of the analysis might influence practitioners and policy makers.

CUA research has seldom, if ever, been subject to such scrutiny. In the United States, decisions to undertake cost-effectiveness research are made by individual investigators, often in conjunction with, or motivated by, government or commercial sponsors. There is little effort to prioritize in order to understand whether we are asking the right questions and focusing on the right problems. Pharmaceutical and device company sponsors often fund economic evaluations to influence reimbursement decisions for their products. These analyses may not be among society's best investments in cost-effectiveness research. In the public sector, there has not been a clearly articulated policy for coordinating CEA research across government agencies. Funding decisions about which areas to favor tend to be made using non-analytical approaches, if they are not at the mercy of the investigators submitting proposals. More coordination and analysis is warranted to define areas in which cost-effectiveness research is likely to have the greatest yield.

11

Advice for Policy Makers and Politicians

. . . .

> *The only way out of this dilemma is for citizens and physicians to accept*
> *the concept and consequences of resource limits, just as they accept speed*
> *limits, zoning laws, and other self-imposed constraints in the interest of the*
> *greater good.*
>
> —Milton Weinstein, 2001

Policy Matters

What should policy makers take away from this book? What can they expect
in the future?

One lesson is that it is important to distinguish resistance to cost-effectiveness analysis on technical grounds from resistance on political grounds.
For the most part, U.S. policy makers haven't attempted to use CEA for
political reasons. The technique hasn't made it to the starting line.

Another lesson is that moving toward cost-effectiveness analysis is a long-
term process that will require changes at several levels. Creating conditions
for its use will take time. Policy makers cannot simply overlay CEA on a
culture and system unprepared for it. Creating the conditions will require
changing the way we think about limits in health care. It will require changing the environment surrounding cost-effectiveness analysis and will involve
various institutional players, from medical journal editors, to government
officials and health plan executives, to judges and juries. This final chapter
considers each in turn.

Institutional Responses

Policy analysts have often wondered why so few health plans in the United
States have funded their own cost-effectiveness analyses, given their complaints

about the studies' poor quality, their skepticism about industry-sponsored studies, and the fact that health plans themselves would be the primary beneficiaries of such analyses (e.g., Reinhardt, 1997; Prosser et al., 2000). To some extent, of course, they have. Some plans have established their own in-house analytical shops (Garber, 2001), while others pay for evaluations of clinical services by groups such as ECRI (Stephenson, 1995). In addition, plans also pay for research and analyses indirectly in many other forms, from journal and newsletter subscriptions to educational seminars.

What has never materialized is the kind of independent body envisioned by many academics over the years; to conduct or evaluate CEAs (e.g., Garrison & Wilensky, 1986; Neumann et al., 1996; Reinhardt, 1997; Lyles, 2001). Reinhardt (1997) has proposed an independent organization for conducting rigorous audits for cost-effectiveness analyses, like those that are standard in financial accounting. Others have drawn from models in the private sector, pointing to organizations providing independent ratings or seals of approval, such as Standard and Poor's (bonds), Underwriters' Laboratories (appliances and electronics), or the National Committee on Quality Assurance (HMOs) (Neumann et al., 1996). Even the editors of the *New England Journal of Medicine*, in the editorial setting down the journal's policy toward CEAs, stated that "if neither the insurance industry nor federal agencies (such as FDA or the Agency for Health Care Policy and Research) are willing or able to fund [cost-effectiveness research], an independent entity funded by a consortium of companies in the drug and device industry could be created expressly to support economic analyses" (Kassirer and Angell, 1994).

Health plans in the United States haven't had to engage in the difficult process of using CEA, according to one line of argument, because they have managed to control costs through more conventional strategies, such as risk-sharing contracts and volume discounts (Litvak et al., 2000). The notion is that once they have reached the limits of containing costs through these other means, they will turn to a CEA as a policy option (Litvak et al., 2000).

Change could come through the benefits language used in insurance contracts. Eddy (1996) has written that "until the idea of cost-effectiveness is accepted as an integral and explicit part of benefit language the country will never solve its cost-quality problem." He has argued for changes in commonly used terms, such as *necessary*, *appropriate*, and *investigational*, to focus instead on health outcomes and cost-effectiveness. And he has proposed adding the term *cost-effective* to benefit language in order to establish its legitimacy, for example, by including the words "an intervention is considered cost-effective if there is no other available intervention that offers a clinically appropriate benefit at a lower cost." But the private health insurance industry—fractious, loath to restrict coverage openly, and already beset by a backlash against its cost-containment practices—has never coalesced around the idea and seems unlikely to do so in the near future.

The pharmaceutical industry, which might support and even fund an independent entity as a way of legitimizing the field they lavishly sponsor, sees more risks than rewards in pursuing such an initiative on its own, fearing that the added costs of doing business would outweigh the benefits. Moreover, the industry has never felt enough external pressure to push for one.

Public officials have also been timid, hamstrung by fears about explicit rationing, and cognizant of the ill-fated experiences of previous U.S. agencies involved in evaluating health technology—from the short-lived National Center for Health Care Technology (Blumenthal, 1983) to the longer-lived but similarly doomed Office of Technology Assessment, which crashed on the shoals of the Republican Congress elected in 1994. The ideological opposition to top-down, bureaucratic, government-run evaluation is strong in Washington. Lobbying groups would be likely to kill any new public agency involved in evaluation.

Public institutions *have* made some progress. As noted, the U.S. Preventive Services Task Force and the U.S. Guide to Community Preventive Services now consider CEA in their recommendations. The initiative has helped us understand how to abstract data for systematic reviews of CEAs and has proven that government efforts can use CEA for certain classes of problems (for example, that focus on preventive services). More concerted action is needed to address what is essentially an information problem. At times, government agencies, such as the Agency for Health Care Research and Quality (AHRQ) and the National Institutes of Health (NIH) have sponsored internal and external research on cost-effectiveness analysis. AHRQ has funded cost-effectiveness research in areas such as lung-volume-reduction surgery, liver transplantation, and heart disease (AHRQ, 2003). NIH has funded studies in cancer, drug-abuse prevention, and other areas (e.g., National Cancer Institute, 2001). Still, the funds devoted to the effort are tiny compared to the amount devoted to basic research. The entire budget for AHRQ in the fiscal year 2002, for example, was approximately $250 million, compared to well over $20 billion for the National Institutes for Health.

There have been formal proposals to increase funding for cost-effectiveness research. For example, proposed legislation in 2003 would have authorized $75 million in annual appropriations—$50 million for NIH and $25 million for AHRQ—to conduct and publish studies on the comparative effectiveness and cost-effectiveness of drugs that account for a high level of expenditures or use by individuals in federally funded health programs (U.S. Congress, HR 2356; Pink Sheet, June 16, 2003). Furthermore, the bill would have required AHRQ to develop standards for the design and conduct of CEAs, and it stipulated that only methodologically sound studies would be considered. The bill was defeated under pressure from the drug industry, however (Pear, 2003). The recently enacted Medicare drug legislation calls for funds for the Agency for Health Care Research and Quality to conduct comparative effectiveness research but explicitly forbids CMS to use the information to withhold coverage of new drugs.

Besides funding, what has never existed is a clearly articulated policy for coordinating CEA research among government agencies. While the federal government conducts or sponsors research in sundry places, it is not directed toward specific decision makers. As noted in chapter 10, there is little effort to prioritize, to understand whether we are asking the right questions and focusing on the right problems. What is done consists of detailed analyses for a few selected clinical strategies, leaving a void for the vast number of strategies whose cost-effectiveness is unknown (Azimi and Welch, 1998).

One option would be to strengthen the FDA, granting the agency authority to examine the cost-effectiveness of prescription drugs in addition to its traditional role of regulating their safety and effectiveness. But changing FDA's mandate in this way would prove to be a mistake. For one thing, FDA lacks the analytical capabilities and the corporate culture to judge cost-effectiveness. More important, diverting the agency's attention from clinical matters toward economic concerns would risk eroding its considerable public support.

A greater role for the Centers for Medicare and Medicaid Services (CMS) would seem natural, particularly in light of the recent Medicare drug benefit legislation. In the future, Congress could also formally consider cost-effectiveness when considering expansion of Medicare-covered services to categories such as disease-management programs, dental services, and vision and hearing services. However, experience has shown the difficulty CMS has had in incorporating cost-effectiveness information explicitly. Even with the new drug benefit, challenges will loom large, perhaps even larger.

Another possible solution would involve creating a new, independent, "NICE-like" agency in the United States. The body could be subsumed as a new agency within the Department of Health and Human Services, or it could even be established as an independent agency within the federal government. But political forces will conspire against it. If created, it would probably become a lightning rod for criticism and its powers stripped.

Officials might instead try to create a quasi-public entity like the Institute of Medicine (IOM) to provide advice for public and private payers. It could conduct its own research or certify that others' evaluations met standards for the field. Such an independent agency could provide the government with valuable advice on the cost-effectiveness of a range of strategies to improve human health. It could also help establish rules for the field and spur a convergence toward good methods. By itself this type of organization would be helpful but still insufficient. Private health plans also need a nimble and more tailored process that can respond to the dynamic world of medical technology innovation and to their own cultures.

The AMCP Format and the Future of Formulary Decision-Making

Formulary submission guidelines such as the Academy of Managed Care Pharmacy (AMCP) Format for Formulary Submissions essentially reproduces—in decentralized, uniquely American fashion—the government processes other countries have implemented to examine the cost-effectiveness of pharmaceuticals (see chapter 8). The growing number of plans using the Format to date suggests that the guidelines are helping fulfill formulary committees' desires for better information. The call for evidence-based formulary decisions, the standardized layout, and the explicit inclusion of information on drugs' value and place in therapy resonate with purchasers. The Format gives plans a flexible but potent management tool to cope with soaring pharmacy bills. Moreover, they permit the kind of "rationing at a distance" that avoids the fallout from more unforgiving forms of cost-containment.

Signs indicate that formulary submission guidelines are here to stay. Though early experience with guidelines have been mixed in terms of the quality and completeness of submissions, drug companies have generally cooperated with the guidelines (Otrompke, 2002). The success the Regence health plan had with a policy under which they refused to review new drugs for the formulary without a full submission from a drug company shows that determined health plans—even small or medium-sized ones—can force pharmaceutical firms to comply (Otrompke, 2002).

Many challenges lie ahead. The precise content and process that emerge will be driven by the plans themselves. Some clinical pharmacists have complained that the Format's prescriptive requirements make dossiers "a phenomenally long and complex process" (Otrompke, 2002). Plans will need to balance the benefits of better information with the costs of implementing new systems.

Over time, the formulary decision makers will determine the nature of the information they want included. They will decide, for example, whether they want the kind of reference case analyses championed by the *Panel*, or other formats that emphasize cost-consequences analyses or budget-impact projections. They will also determine the degree to which they are willing to tolerate deviations from the Format's requirements; for economic models, off-label information, full disclosure of funding sources, and information on indirect or productivity costs. And they will need to address the degree to which plans want analyses using their own data and how to ensure the confidentiality of pharmaceutical submissions.

A corollary benefit of the Format may be the production of cost-effectiveness analyses that pay greater attention to "real-world" impacts. These include the effects on complication rates, adherence to drug regimens, and settings of care (Pignone et al., 2002; Tunis et al., 2003).

In the end, the process will probably also drive institutional rearrangements to address the inefficiencies of maintaining what would, in effect, be hundreds of local NICE-like bodies requesting dossiers and duplicating one another's efforts. Instead, a few large pharmaceutical benefits managers might set up a "super-AMCP Format" process, for example, and disseminate information to subscribing plans. Alternatively, a consortium of private plans may create their own evaluative body. The group of states working with the State of Oregon to share the costs and use the results of evidence-based reviews demonstrates that this process has begun in the public sector as well (Kaiser Commission on Medicaid and the Uninsured, 2004). Pharmaceutical companies, for their part, will probably produce a single, flexible dossier that can be tailored to the needs of individual plans.

What the Courts May Do

An important, lingering question is how the courts will view cost-effectiveness analysis. Jacobson and Kanna (2001) note that if the medical profession begins to accept cost-effectiveness analysis as an input into standards of care, the courts could incorporate the information by deferring to professional custom. These authors argue that as long as analyses are conducted by qualified experts using standard methods, cost-effectiveness evidence should be admissible, though they caution that it should be viewed as *one* piece of evidence for a jury to consider and not by itself set the standard of care. They draw a parallel to how courts have viewed clinical guidelines (see Brennan, 1991; Rosoff, 2001; Jacobson and Kanna, 2001).

In the future, courts might react on a case-by-case basis to establish whether and how CEA should be incorporated into standard of care (Jacobson and Kanna, 2001).[1] To some extent this may already be happening, as national bodies such as the U.S. Task Force on Preventive Services (Saha et al., 2001) and other organizations incorporate cost-effectiveness information (Wallace et al., 2002).

As far as institutional capacity is concerned, Jacobson and Kanna (2001) note that judges may retain outside experts and assess analyses to determine the admissibility of cost-effectiveness evidence, though juries would weigh that evidence once admitted. This could create the impetus to develop the clarity, transparency, pre-specification, and commitment to empirical evidence from the courts that some have called for (Eddy, 2001).

Another potential strategy involves working through Medicare/Medicaid managed care to introduce cost-effectiveness analysis, and then allowing courts to develop a standard of care that defers to congressional policy regarding CEA (Jacobson and Kanna, 2001). In this way cost-effectiveness analysis could migrate to nongovernmental programs and avoid the "smoking gun" problem. Jacobson and Kanna (2001) argue that "in view of the Supreme Court's strong endorsement of managed care's cost containment strategies, this approach seems plausible."

Change could also come in managed-care contracts, which might more explicitly specify covered and uncovered services, and also define how and when cost-effectiveness would be used (Havighurst, 1995; Hall, 1997; Studdert and Gresenz, 2002). Medical directors surveyed recently stated that clearer cost-effectiveness criteria and evidence could improve the utility of contractual definitions (Singer and Gergthold, 2001). Health insurers in the future might bargain to include CEA in the health benefits contract, which could specify processes for patient appeals and include information on the implications for subscribers. Health insurance contracts could appeal to evidence from CEAs—for example, as a basis for limiting mammogram coverage for women under 50, or use it as part of the basis of medical necessity determinations (Jacobson and Kanna, 2001).

To avoid a smoking gun, plans could bring the public into the decision-making process and make their criteria for covering services much more clear and explicit (Jacobson and Kanna, 2001). Eddy (2001) has argued that plans should give explicit descriptions of the standard of evidence that will be used to determine coverage and the role that costs and cost-effectiveness analysis will play in the process. He believes that plans should be clear about what type of coverage they offer, that people should be free to choose among coverage options, and that courts should hold parties to their commitments.

Yet each of these recommendations raises problems. It seems more likely that health plans will continue to shield themselves from suits by avoiding explicit policies that put them in a position of denying coverage based on costs. As Studdert and Gresenz (2002) note, "purchasers' distaste for explicit rationing, together with apprehension about incomprehensible road maps of covered benefits, have traditionally chilled interest in a more prescriptive approach to coverage." As a result, discussions about regulatory interventions designed to protect consumers are primarily concerned with ensuring that the *processes* that health plans use to decide questions of coverage are fair, prompt, careful, and subject to review, rather than explaining issues of cost-effectiveness (Studdert and Gresenz, 2002).

Moreover, even if they could be convinced of the importance of cost-effectiveness considerations, plans would continue to worry about how juries will respond. In the future, judges could provide explicit instructions to juries on how to weigh CEA evidence, what role CEA plays in setting the standard of care, and the fact that it is entirely appropriate for plans and physicians to consider CEA (Jacobson and Kanna, 2001). But this would be likely to prove dangerous legal ground for plans to tread. While CEA in theory could benefit either plaintiffs or defendants, plaintiffs might be the likelier beneficiaries if—as Hastie and Viscusi (1998) argue—jurors exhibit hindsight bias (people overestimate *ex ante* risks and underestimate *ex ante* benefits): when confronted *ex post* with real-life victims, jurors overestimate the risks that victims face compared to the *ex ante* hypothetical case. In the end, using CEA may expose the classical divide problem of underemphasizing statistical lives and overemphasizing identifiable lives.

As far as the idea of Medicare's working through the regulatory system to incorporate CEA, given the agency's inability to even broach the matter explicitly and the strong resistance this approach would be likely to encounter in the political arena, it seems improbable.

Regarding contracts, consumers do not usually negotiate over contractual terms. There are practical limits on the details specified in contracts, and existing evidence is often of insufficient scientific quality in any event. Moreover, the vast majority of contractual coverage appeals involve items such as durable medical equipment (e.g., foot orthotics), ancillary health services, physical therapy, dental care, alternative medicine, infertility treatments, and investigational/experimental treatments (Studdert and Gresenz, 2002), which are not typically subject to formal cost-effectiveness analysis.

In the end, the best way for plans to interact with the courts with respect to CEA is to stay out of them (Eddy, 2001). Plans might view the AMCP Format as a desirable strategy in this regard because it provides a firmer basis for considering evidence while avoiding potentially damaging explicit CEA policies—especially if CEA is used merely as one input for determining a drug's status as "preferred" or "non-preferred," rather than rejecting it outright. Courts have traditionally deferred to plans' cost-containment strategies and would probably continue to defer, as long as the courts could just ensure that fair process was established and that CEA was not applied in a capricious manner (Jacobson and Kanna, 2001).

Lessons from Abroad

What can U.S. policy makers learn from their counterparts abroad? On the one hand, different values and cultures make drawing parallels hazardous. Cross-national surveys reveal greater support overseas for government health programs and less concern about having access to the latest technologies (Blendon et al., 1990; Kim et al., 2001). The willingness to use CEA as an explicit policy tool in many countries reflects these proclivities. The emergence of the National Institute of Clinical Excellence (NICE) in the United Kingdom, for example, was predicated on the strong British tradition in public health, as well as other factors such as the evidence-based medicine culture and the country's stable of health economics and outcomes researchers (Akehurst, 2001).

Still, U.S. policy makers should watch these experiences closely. They prove that, given the right political circumstances, public officials can apply cost-effectiveness analysis openly. They confirm that the United States's failure to use CEA is driven more by its own cultural conditions than by the technique's inherent methodological shortcomings.

In many countries, CEA has forced a more careful consideration of available evidence (Sculpher et al., 2001). It has motivated decision makers to ask the right questions about what evidence is relevant, which services are "best practice," how good the intermediate outcomes measures are, how valid the data collection instruments are, and how much uncertainty exists (Sculpher et al., 2001; Cookson, 2000; Mitchell, 2002).

The Australian experience has revealed that formal review by authorities can detect problems of interpretation not found even in top peer-reviewed journals (Cookson, 2000; Mitchell, 2002). NICE has shown that the process can help target funding by illuminating the consequences of directing resources to particular patient subgroups or strategies.

The international experiences have also demonstrated a kind of rough triumph for cost-effectiveness thresholds. In Australia, a threshold between $42K and $76K per life year (AUS) has emerged (George et al., 2001). In the United Kingdom, despite the government's official denials, a threshold of £30/K atr QALY seems to hold at NICE, except for "special cases" such as drugs for multiple sclerosis. (While the United Kingdom's Department of Health's own circular says that NICE has not adopted a standard threshold, it admits that "retrospective analysis suggests positive recommendations associated with cost per QALY of £30K . . . and that "high cost/QALY figures have been accepted only if there were special factors . . . not covered by the formal modeling" (Towse and Pritchard, 2002)).

Even these special cases prove the value of the process. In the case of drugs for multiple sclerosis (MS), NICE's own experts said the medications were not cost-effective in terms of cost per QALYs, but political pressures prevailed upon authorities to make treatment available for patients with this life-threatening disease (Taylor, 2001). The cost-effectiveness analysis helped to establish the boundaries for the debate and to inform the ultimate resolution, which involved giving patients access to the medications but placing drug companies at financial risk if the patients declined more rapidly than predicted by the company's models—a solution described as a way to secure therapy for patients "in a manner that could be considered cost-effective" (Taylor, 2001). As its staunchest proponents would have it, CEA provided a structured process of evaluating the strength of evidence, stating assumptions, and forcing a discussion of the service's value, all of which brought insight that was as helpful in its way as the final C/E estimates themselves (Gold et al., 1996). The MS case also demonstrated that the evaluation process was flexible when circumstances warranted it.

The British process has also revealed pitfalls. Expectations for a CEA policy need to be realistic and not be oversold.

NICE created a fat political target. It could be argued that this is a positive outcome; that it has forced an explicit debate about the tradeoffs society must confront and the ethical judgments underlying CEAs. Smith (2000) observes that NICE "had to exist in order for us to begin to think about something better."

U.S. policy makers need to understand and anticipate the controversy that NICE has provoked, however. The creation of NICE generated a round of criticism about explicit rationing rather than the consideration of how much in overall resources the National Health Service (NHS) should provide for health care (Towse and Pritchard, 2002).

NICE has also created another regulatory step for manufacturers (the "fourth hurdle"), which could impede innovation and delay access to new treatments. The Australian Pharmaceutical Manufacturers Association has argued, for example, that time to market increased by six months in the wake of the country's cost-effectiveness provision for new pharmaceuticals, though an Australian National Audit Office study found no increased administrative delays in the submission process (Cookson, 2000).

Moreover, explicit considerations of cost-effectiveness may not save money. In Australia, drug spending grew after cost-effectiveness evidence was required for pharmaceutical submissions in 1992 and has accelerated in recent years (Mitchell, 2002). Recommendations by NICE have tended to "level up" access to pharmaceuticals (Taylor, 2001). While proponents of CEA are fond of saying that the technique is not designed to save money but to target resources more efficiently, the political calculation changes when the new policy comes with a higher price tag, especially when its application—and the term *cost-effectiveness* itself—seems to promise cost savings.

Considering cost-effectiveness also requires resources for implementation. Evidence costs money. It also requires a new bureaucracy. Poor-quality submissions in Australia highlight the need for sophistication at the reviewer level (Cookson, 2000). Without it, technical problems will persist in methodology, transparency, and accountability.

And even with resources, an agency armed with CEA can only do so much. Only a fraction of services are ever subject to rigorous evaluation. Many decisions with huge spending implications, such as the closure of hospital beds for the elderly and mentally ill and substituting care in the community (Akehurst, 2001), are introduced without evaluation in cost or outcome terms. Raferty (2001) has reported that the net cost of implementing the NICE recommendations were around £200m, less than 0.5% of annual spending on NHS. Most of NICE's attention has been focused on pharmaceuticals, though they only account for 12% of NHS spending (Akehurst, 2001).

CEA and the Medicare Program

To Medicare, CEA has been an elephant in the living room, officially ignored despite its obvious importance. After a decade of failed attempts to integrate CEA as a criterion for coverage, prospects for its ultimate adoption at the time of this writing appear dim.

These attempts have revealed the strength of antagonism in the U.S. towards openly confronting resource constraints. If Medicare officials—and politicians—learned anything from the experience, it was the political folly of trying to ration honestly.

Despite soaring health costs, there is no apparent reason to believe this sentiment will change. Even Medicare's latest, watered-down attempt to define the criteria it would use in covering new technologies—one that proposed a narrow consideration of costs, and only in situations where competing technology offered equivalent benefits (*U.S. Federal Register*, 2000)—has proven politically unacceptable. Physicians are already angered and frustrated by Centers for Medicare and Medicaid Services. Medicare is popular with the public and with beneficiaries, and policymakers and politicians will not risk being tagged as jeopardizing it. Moreover, the CMS is currently preoccupied with a host of other challenges, including major new statutory provisions and responsibilities to regulate private health insurance and implement electronic data standards (Iglehart, 2002).

At the same time, Medicare cannot avoid difficult decisions about costly new technology. What's a $400 billion agency to do?

Most likely it will stumble along, evading the tough choices by relegating authority to private health plans and cutting payment rates, and by allowing incentives in the system to dictate actual utilization. Costly new technology that offers positive health benefits will be covered, but its use will be determined by prevailing payment policy.

The criteria used to determine coverage are critical. Creation of the Medicare Coverage Advisory Committee (MCAC) was a positive step forward and signaled a greater commitment to clinical evidence, as well as created a more transparent and understandable coverage process for medical technology. It provides the kind of broad and independent scientific expertise that CMS needs. CMS now provides a public tracking system and publishes coverage decisions as decision memos, for example. Final decisions are more clearly labeled: "full coverage," "coverage with limitations," "noncoverage," "coverage at discretion of regional contractors. "There is greater opportunity for public input."

MCAC also took a small but important step toward determining the value of medical services. It set a precedent of first establishing the adequacy of evidence about the intervention's effectiveness in routine clinical use among Medicare beneficiaries, and then considering the magnitude of benefit (Garber, 2001).

Still, the effort has fallen short. For one thing, given the reach of its decisions, the MCAC remains a woefully small operation, with annual costs of about $700,000 for compensation and travel expenses of members, and 5.5 annual person-years of staff at a cost of $359,790 (HCFA, 2001).

More important, rules for determining the magnitude of benefit remain vague.[2] CMS is effectively not permitted to debate the relative costs of new services given the benefits conferred. A new technology that offers modest benefits even at enormous additional expense will presumably be covered, with no debate about its relative value.

With one hand tied behind its back, the best that CMS can do at the moment is to work around the constraint and endeavor to be a prudent purchaser, even while publicly professing its opposition to restrictions and its desire to ensure access to important advances. In part the juggling act will involve crafting acceptable language. In a sense, CMS needs to develop "code" words for cost-effectiveness.

Medicare officials have already used the term *comparability* in this way. HCFA Administrator Nancy Ann DeParle, in a statement before Congress in 1998 (DeParle, March, 12, 1998), stated that the criteria used to guide coverage decisions on whether service is reasonable and necessary are: (1) demonstrated effectiveness; (2) appropriateness; and (3) *comparability* to similar services. DeParle defined "demonstrated effectiveness" as follows: "authoritative evidence must demonstrate that the benefits of a service or technology will result in improved patient management or health outcomes, such as decreased morbidity or mortality."[3] She defined "appropriateness" to mean that the service must be suitable for the beneficiary's needs and condition, performed by qualified personnel in suitable settings. In outlining *comparability*, she gave the purest expression of Medicare crypto-speak, denying that Medicare would ever use cost-effectiveness for purposes of coverage, even while establishing its precedent for guiding payment policy:

> Finally, if a service is an alternative or a replacement for a currently covered service, we consider how this new service compares with such other service. The purpose of this comparison is to address payment rather than coverage issues. *Let me be clear: HCFA does not and will not refuse to cover a service because it is costly.* Nevertheless, as a prudent purchaser of health care, if a service is an alternative or a replacement for a currently-covered service for the same diagnostic or therapeutic purpose, HCFA will examine both the relative costs and effectiveness in determining what Medicare payment policy should be. For example, if a new service is more expensive but equally effective as the currently-covered service, it would still be covered but paid at a rate of the lower cost alternative. If, however, the service is found to be

more effective, it would be paid at the higher rate. This criterion assures that the Medicare program and its beneficiaries receive the best value" [italics added].

CMS tried to codify this policy in its May 2000 Notice, stating that "we believe that by comparing two items or services that are included in a Medicare benefit category, we increase beneficiary access and add value to the program" (HCFA, May 16, 2000). It added that, "In particular, if a new item or service is equivalent in benefit, is in the same clinical modality, is thus substitutable for the existing service, and is lower in costs, we would consider withdrawing coverage for the more expensive currently covered alternative service. . . ." It further qualified: "since we anticipate limiting the application of costs to a narrower situation when two services have equivalent health outcomes and are of the same clinical modality, we need to do only a simple cost-analysis" (*U.S. Federal Register*, 2000–31128). As noted earlier, this Notice never advanced into formal policy.

In some difficult cases, Medicare might develop "limited coverage" when a service depends on the skills of practitioners (Buto, 1994), or "coverage with conditions," essentially the approach used for coverage of trial costs associated with lung-volume-reduction surgery. As Administrator Vladeck noted, conditional coverage "may be used when existing data suggest a potential benefit to some patients, but there is not sufficient information to predict the effect of generalized use of the technology or its long term effects or appropriate patient selection criteria." He added that the goal was to "advance medical knowledge about the effectiveness of the services before they are diffused to general practice and to assure that Medicare beneficiaries are not put at undue risk from their use" (U.S. Congress, 1997). This is not cost-effectiveness but a way to address fiscal issues while maintaining access for some patients. Application of this provision would presumably be limited to difficult cases where benefits are unproven.

All of this discussion anticipates implementation of the new Medicare drug benefit. Many questions remain about how decisions about new drugs for Medicare beneficiaries will be made in practice. But a key question will involve the criteria used to determine coverage for new drugs. The history of Medicare suggests that it will be difficult, if not impossible, for the program to use CEA explicitly in this process, at least centrally on the national level.

CEA might be used instead by private plans who administer the benefit. Plans and PBMs could adopt an AMCP-like process, which allows decision makers to consider the cost-effectiveness of new drugs more explicitly.

Overly restrictive formularies could produce a backlash, however, and the process will need to be handled delicately.

Take-Home Lessons

Ever-rising health spending, the inexorable march of new drugs and other technologies, improvements in analytical methods, and the trend overseas to use economic evaluation explicitly in coverage decisions, all produce momentum for CEA in the United States.

At the same time political realities will continue to intrude. If anything, signals from the recent past point to a growing backlash *against* the imposition of limits. As Robinson (2001) has noted, protagonists of managed care have been in full retreat, broadening physician panels, removing restrictions, and reverting to fee-for-service payments. Widespread skepticism of government, corporate, and professional dominance has fueled consumerism, and forced government entities to avoid politically volatile initiatives to balance the allocation of limited resources.

In this climate, there is unlikely to be a groundswell for CEA, despite the larger forces. Despite predictions that administrators and policy makers will become better at using CEA (Ubel, 2000), the technique is unlikely to ascend quickly as a policy-making tool.

Instead, health insurers and employers will continue to impose limits in other ways; for example, by creating incentives for individuals to become more cost-conscious consumers of health care. We can expect public and private payers to increase cost-sharing levels, implement tiered benefits for prescription drugs and even hospitals and physician networks, and experiment with defined contributions, rather than defined benefits (Toner and Stahlberg, 2002; Center for Health Systems Change, 2002).

Politically, it will probably remain easier to impose limits by restricting eligibility rather than services, or by not providing coverage at all (Vladeck, 2000). The great irony of the American health system—that we spend enormous sums of money but don't cover everyone—will endure.

The more plausible scenario is one in which coverage decisions reflect an untidy combination of evidence- and politics-based medicine, and in which CEA plays a supporting role. This is not entirely a bad thing. Policy makers need to respect the democratic process, even as they strive to maximize health with society's limited resources (Singer, 1997). But policy makers can also learn from experience a number of important take-home lessons about CEA.

CEA should not be used rigidly

Leaders in the field have always warned against using CEA rigidly, but it took the Oregon plan's misadventures to drive home the lesson. That experience should dissuade others from attempting to use CEA in mechanical fashion. The Oregon experience should also caution policy makers to lower expectations in the first place. As Mitchell (2002) has observed about the Australian experience, objectives for CEA should be modest, particularly in early stages. Policy makers should tread cautiously, and not adhere to the notion that there is a single solution. Rather, CEA should first gain a stronger foothold by winning smaller successes (e.g., in the selective use of CEA by developers of clinical guidelines).

Cost-effectiveness analysis is likely to prove more acceptable if applied to preventive services rather than treatment for acute care because it doesn't involve patients who are already ill. Decision makers may find CEA most helpful as an aid for making comparisons between interventions within a particular illness or condition, such as the most cost-effective way to treat cancer (Earle et al., 2000) or cardiovascular disease (Winkelmeyer et al., 2003). Eddy (1996) recommends using cost-effectiveness in this context for benefit language, advising that health plans adopt language stipulating that "the intervention is the most cost-effective method available to address the medical condition. . . ."

CEA does not mean cost containment

A second lesson is that CEA should not be promoted as a cost-containment tool. Instead, it should be thought of as a technique for obtaining better value, not a way to eliminate services but a way to target resources more efficiently.

Implementation of a CEA policy is not likely to save money. Indeed, the opposite is likely to be true. Where policy makers have implemented CEA, health costs have risen. By shedding light on the value of services provided, one is more likely to reveal under- rather than over-treatment.[4] But CEA can help target resources to efficient uses to help ensure that society is receiving optimal health for its investments.

Separate evaluation from payment

An important institutional lesson is that those evaluating cost-effectiveness evidence should be separated from those making coverage or payment decisions. Evaluators should provide independent analyses and maintain a healthy distance from the political forces confronting decision makers. Moreover, their recommendations should not be binding, a policy followed by most international technology assessment organizations. The arrangement allows evaluators a measure of protection in conducting their inquiries. It also takes some heat off payers, who can appeal to findings from independent evaluators.

NICE provides an example of the arrangement. It is a health authority of NHS and a quasi-government institution. The NICE appraisal committee is chosen for technical competence, but it doesn't actually pay for care (NHS does, with payment through taxation). The review of evidence is separated from policy making (Akehurst, 2001).

How you say it matters

Physicians understand that resources are limited. They accept the need to contain costs and even believe that individual physicians should play role in considering cost-effectiveness. Many of the physicians interviewed in one survey stated that they sometimes discussed costs or cost-effectiveness with patients (Sacramento Health Care, 2001). At the same time, physicians are not willing to admit to rationing (Ubel, 2000).

Similarly, health-plan managers deny that they ration care but admit that their budgets are constrained, and that cost is a factor in decision making (Prosser et al., 2000). More than half of medical directors surveyed in one study stated that they would consider a less costly, equally effective intervention before a more costly one in making a coverage decision about a new intervention (Singer and Bergthold, 2001).

These responses are instructive. They suggest that the term *cost-effectiveness* may be part of the problem. Insisting on an "eat your broccoli" approach—that Americans must simply come to grips with the need to ration—is unlikely to work.

The term *cost-effectiveness* has taken on an unappealing cast. Policy makers need to use language that conveys a sense of fairness and hope, rather than limits. Researchers and policy makers would do well to search for ways to communicate the information in more acceptable fashion. Various options outlined earlier include using the terms *value analysis* or *comparability*.

Process matters

A key take-home lesson is the importance of procedural issues surrounding the application of CEA. Medical ethicists have written about the importance of *fair process*, especially when citizens can't agree on the underlying distributive principles, or even about what constitutes a fair outcome. How to successfully apply CEA is in part a procedural question: establishing the conditions for public deliberation and democratic oversight of priority-setting in health care (Daniels and Sabin, 2002).

What constitutes fair process? As Daniels and Sabin (2002) ask, "under what conditions should society grant authority to individuals or institutions to set limits to health care?" They cite four necessary conditions that they argue characterize key features of fair process:

- *Publicity*: decisions (e.g., coverage or drug formulary decisions) and the rationale for making them must be publicly accessible;
- *Relevance*: there must be a reasonable explanation for a decision's rationale that is acceptable by fair-minded people;
- *Revision and appeals*: decisions must be subject to revision and appeal;
- *Regulative:* some voluntary or public regulation of the process must ensure the first three conditions are met.

Daniel and Sabin (2002) think that the successful application of these criteria would address the legitimacy problem. Publicity, they argue, would establish more efficient, coherent, and fairer decisions over time and strengthen broader public deliberations. Similar individuals would be treated similarly, or if situations demand a different rationale, the circumstances or principles would be known. The relevance condition would ensure that decisions are not "bureaucratically arbitrary," or based on reasons that people don't view as meaningful or just, and would invite a conversation with stakeholders. The appeals condition would provide a mechanism for challenge and change, which contributes to democratic governance (and helps avoid courts, which are not good places to argue about details of clinical evidence). The regulative condition ensures enforcement of the process.

Can policy makers apply these conditions to address CEA's legitimacy problem? Reasons for pessimism are easy to cite. Grounds for coverage decisions are not routinely made public. Health plans typically do not provide the rationale underlying their decisions. Appeals processes vary considerably. A view seems to prevail among government and corporate leaders that publicity for CEA will not work in the United States because of fear of litigation and media exposure; that the costs of openness outweigh the benefits.

The counter-argument is that we have never really tried it, that there is little evidence to show that disseminating reasons for decisions has actually made organizations more vulnerable to bad press or litigation (Daniels and Sabin, 2002). The possibility remains that openness would actually provide the best protections against such charges. Some legal analysts believe that courts would defer to the stated practice of health plans as long as an appropriate process was followed (Jacobson and Kanna, 2001). It is at least plausible to believe that public trust would go *up*, not down, if consumers were involved in designing the process and if the process were more transparent. Tensions might best be allayed by open deliberation about the fair terms of cooperation. The public might display far more reasonableness than politicians give them credit for.

There are even some signs of progress. Fair process has emerged as a key issue in the debates over rights to sue managed-care plans, for example. Some plans are working to spur consumer participation in the design of insurance, the patient grievance process, and coverage decisions (Sacramento Health Care, 2001). Some large HMOs have made treatment guidelines public, posting the information on their websites, and even publicizing how they pay doctors, including the financial incentives for physicians (Freudenheim, 2003).[5] Medicare has moved towards more openness in its coverage process. None of these initiatives has involved CEA, however, though at least one survey has detected a willingness among consumers to accept physicians' use of CEA as one treatment criterion, especially if they trust that the physician's opinion not coerced or financially rewarded, or if made by unbiased medical experts (Sacramento Health Care, 2001).

The National Institute of Clinical Excellence in the United Kingdom illustrates the possibilities of including CEA in an open manner. NICE now publishes information on its website at several stages, including scope of appraisal, literature review, provisional views, and draft guidance (Mayor, 2002). Institute staff hold meetings with stakeholder groups, including relevant patient organizations, doctors, and pharmaceutical companies. NICE officials point to the case of imatinib (Gleevec) as an example of the flexibility of the process (Mayor, 2002). NICE first announced that it would only cover the drug for patients in the accelerated phase of disease, but then changed its recommendation based on the input of external organizations to include other groups of patients (e.g., those in the chronic phase as well, those for whom interferon alpha had failed or who could not tolerate it). The NICE chairman has publicly spoken about the importance of being as open as possible (Mayor, 2002).

Raise the threshold

The commonly used benchmark of $50,000/QALY to reflect society's willingness to pay for health benefits has murky origins. Most commonly, researchers point to Medicare's decision in the 1970s to cover dialysis for patients with chronic renal failure, which at the time had a C/E ratio in this range and thus created a convenient yardstick for the field (Gold et al., 1996; Ubel, Hirth et al., 2003). Occasionally, analysts use an upper boundary of $100,000 for a threshold of what society should deem affordable (Winkelmeyer and Neumann, 2002). More recently, many cost-effectiveness investigators have justified their conclusion about what is affordable by citing a 1992 paper by Laupacis et al., which claimed that interventions with a C/E ratio under Can$20K are attractive options, those in the range of Can$20,000 to Can$100,000 comprise possibly cost-effective interventions; and those above Can$100,000 reflect unfavorable investments (Winkelmeyer and Neumann, 2002).

Judging the appropriate threshold presents an ongoing challenge. As Ubel and colleagues (2003) point out, the threshold should be compatible with multiple societal goals—it would need to *decrease* over time if society wanted to constrain health costs. Whether society could afford to pay for every additional intervention that cost, say, $100,000/QALY is highly questionable. Moreover, as noted throughout this book, the use of a single, universally applicable threshold creates problems; actual willingness to pay for health gains depends on the context of the problem and the perspective of decision makers.

Evidence from various quarters suggests that the existing threshold is too low. For one thing, the dialysis example is decades old. If society were willing to spend $50,000 for each QALY gained 20 years ago, shouldn't we be willing to spend more for one now? Even the often cited Lapaucis et al. benchmark is a decade old. Furthermore, analysts rarely account for inflation over time, nor do they convert from Canadian to U.S. dollars (Winkelmeyer and Neumann, 2002).

Evidence from the "statistical value-of-life literature," which uses willingness-to-pay (WTP) surveys and revealed-preference approaches to infer the value of a life from actual behavior (i.e., an individual's willingness to accept higher pay to compensate for riskier jobs) suggests a value of $265,000 per QALY (in 1997 dollars) (Hirth et al., (2000)). Hirth and colleagues (2000) found that, of 35 statistical value-of-life studies, 28 had WTP amounts of over $100,000. Therefore, the threshold should probably be raised, though monitored and revisited, particularly with respect to how use of a higher threshold influences behavior.

Incentives first

Debates about the use of cost-effectiveness should never be divorced from debates about the underlying health-care system. One of the chief complaints against NICE is not about CEA per se, but about a single organization's being in charge of making recommendations about value. How CEA's will be employed in the U.S. health system—whether centrally by CMS, for example, or decentrally by competing PBMs—will be a critical issue in the future.

The drug industry's opposition to Medicare's use of cost-effectiveness has more to do with "big government" than with the technique as such. PhRMA has written, "Cost-effectiveness analysis in the private sector can provide useful information. When employed by centralized decision-makers, however, it often becomes just another term for health care rationing . . . in the private sector the effects are mitigated by plurality of health insurers" (PhRMA letter, 2003).

The incentives inherent in any health system will continue to play a great role in determining the use of services, regardless of whether policy makers use CEA. Most rationing by physicians will still be performed in response to incentives or disincentives provided by third-party payers (Levinsky, 1998). Making consumers and physicians more cost-conscious decision makers is critical.

In the United Kingdom there is explicit consideration of CEA, but other incentives in the system play a large role in determining the services that are actually used. Tight budgets at the physician practice and primary-care-trust (groups of practices) level, as well as an explicit profit control mechanism that affects the price of drugs, loom large in determining use.

Realignment of incentives is a precondition for the successful application of CEA. Weinstein (2001) has argued for changes in the incentives facing physicians so that they act in the collective interest. He notes that expecting physicians to consider cost-effectiveness analysis at the bedside places them in an untenable position as agents for two sometimes adversarial principals: the individual patient and the larger community. A physician responsible for a collection of patients and faced with a resource budget or accountable for the resources he consumes could be put in a situation similar to that of an emergency room physician performing triage. In theory the physician could be responsible for setting or implementing priorities and could invoke CEA data to guide priorities—for example, considering incremental health benefits, and having the flexibility to give added moral consideration to applying resources to the most desperate cases.

Think broadly across sectors

There is a strong, long-standing case that the United States could achieve more protection against public health and environmental risks at less over-all cost to society if priorities were determined or influenced by the insights of CEA (Harvard Group on Risk Management, 1995; Graham, 1996). Tengs and Graham (1996) estimated that 60,000 lives could be saved by reallo-cating investments across medical, public health, and environmental life-saving interventions, from those with high cost-effectiveness ratios to those with low ratios.

The figure has been criticized both on technical grounds and on grounds that broad allocations across sectors (e.g., from environmental health to medicine) are infeasible (Heinzerling and Ackerman, 2002). But the esti-mates illustrates the power of thinking broadly about the way society allo-cates resources for health care.

Often, rankings of cost-effectiveness ratios have only focused on a single disease area, such as cancer (e.g., Earle et al., 2000) or HIV (Pinkerton et al., 2001); less often have they been used in broader societal perspective ex-plicitly (Jamison et al., 1993; Hutubessy et al., 2002). John Graham, formerly a professor at the Harvard School of Public Health, long ago called for more rational, science-based priority setting at the federal level, to subject new regulations to cost-benefit analysis, and to use cost-effectiveness analy-sis to ensure that investments were being made efficiently. He pointed out that at least 12 federal agencies have statutory responsibility for regulating risks. The largest is EPA, and the others include FDA, the Occupational Safety and Health Administration, and the National Highway Traffic Safety Administration (Graham, 1996).

Graham's elevation to Administrator of the Office of Information and Regulatory Affairs at the Office of Management and Budget raised the profile of cost-effectiveness analysis and the potential for incorporating formal analysis into policy (AEI-Brookings, 2001). The fiscal year 2003 federal budget (http://www.whitehouse.gov/omb/inforeg/spec24.pdf) describes steps OMB is taking toward the increased use of CEA to evaluate regulations across a broad range of regulatory sectors. That document also lists CEA estimates that OMB has developed based on analyses released by various agencies.

In its draft 2003 report to Congress on the costs and benefits of major health and safety regulations, OMB called for improving the technical quality of benefit-cost estimates and expanding methods to embrace cost-effectiveness analysis as well as cost-benefit analysis in regulatory decisions. While the report does not favor cost-benefit analysis over cost-effectiveness analysis, it does encourage agencies to do both because they offer somewhat different but useful perspectives. OMB notes, for example, that cost-effectiveness analyses are most helpful for comparing sets of regulatory actions with same primary outcome (U.S. Office of Management and Budget, 2003).

The need for leadership

John Kitzhaber, the architect of the Oregon plan, has remarked that political pressures on the system serve to make sure no one denies anybody benefits (cited in Goldsmith, 2003). To forge any kind of consensus on cost-effectiveness in this environment, leadership will be needed at local, state, and federal levels to frame the debate and to push for legislative changes where necessary.

At this time, it seems unlikely that the United States will muster the political will needed to create an agency resembling the United Kingdom's National Institute for Clinical Excellence. But changes in other public institutions, such as NIH, AHRQ, CDC, and EPA, are beginning to promote the value of cost-effectiveness at a tool to guide prioritization.

Changing public attitudes is the most formidable challenge of all. A prevailing view is that Americans will not accept limits in their use of health care. But society's notion of limits changes when the cost of *not* addressing them becomes excessive. Over time, we have imposed constraints on once-impenetrable redoubts of liberty. We have banned smoking, required seatbelts, made motorcyclists wear helmets, and imposed speed limits on our highways. All of these changes required evidence to support their merits and strong leaders to introduce legislation and convince the public that the benefits exceeded their costs. As health costs grow at unsustainable rates, we will find ways to impose limits in this area as well.

Conclusions

In the end, the use of CEA in the United States to date gets a decidedly mixed review. Improvements in the analytical approach and advances in its applications have been checked by strong political opposition.

The energetic push toward evidence-based medicine shows that coverage and reimbursement decisions cannot be derived from evidence alone. Even with backing by solid clinical evidence, decisions about how we spend our health-care resources demand judgments about how much we are willing to forego in other areas to achieve improvements in health.

A body of research has shed light on the roots of opposition to CEA. Evidence shows that it has to do with unfamiliarity with the methods, mistrust of practitioners' motives and above all a deep-seated public unease with the technique as a tool for rationing. The manner in which U.S. policy makers have addressed and resisted CEA highlights, in considerable relief, entrenched instincts among Americans: mistrust of government, inclination towards market solutions, antipathy for solutions that impose restrictions.

CEA has never occupied the place at the health policy table that many experts had anticipated. Twenty-five years after its promotion to the medical community, it still suffers from a fundamental problem of legitimacy. Proponents of cost-effectiveness analysis have never really confronted these sentiments. Instead, their tendency has been to criticize the existing situation and simply wait with a detached sense of inevitability for soaring health spending to force Americans to do what appeals to reason could not.

My goal in this book was for a finer resolution of the matter. Opposition to CEA as a limit-setting technique cannot be denied or wished away. History shows that the wait for the inevitable may take considerable time.

Where is the United States in 2004 on this issue? More important, where will we be in 2014 or 2024? Are we perched at the beginning of a long social learning curve, where, say, Norway or the United Kingdom were 10 or 20 years ago, or are we off the curve altogether on our own American trajectory, destined to sidestep the problem and confront our limits through other means: imposing cost-sharing arrangements, hassling patients who attempt to get costly health services, and tolerating the fact that one-sixth of our population lives without health insurance?

At this juncture, the smart betting would be on the latter. There seems no reason to believe that major social change is on the horizon.

But this book ends on a note of optimism for CEA. I believe the United States has already begun its precarious journey on the long social learning curve. We may never be at peace with the principle of living within our means. We may fiercely strive to receive expensive new medical technologies that offer any health benefits. But we will find ways to compromise. And we will find ways to use cost-effectiveness analysis in a more explicit fashion than we do today.

Notes

. . . .

Chapter 2

1. Leading methodological journals publishing CUAs in this period included: *Pharmacoeconomics* (28), *International Journal of Technology Assessment in Health Care* (18), and *Medical Decision Making* (13).

2. Clinical journals in the top 15 included *AIDS*, the *American Journal of Medicine*, *Circulation*, *Journal of Clinical Oncology*, *Journal of Vascular Surgery*, *Journal of General Internal Medicine*, *Stroke*, *Radiology*, and *Transfusion*.

Chapter 3

1. Drugs and biologics that meet Medicare program requirements have traditionally been covered by Medicare if they are FDA approved. In addition, off-label indications of these products can be approved if they are considered generally accepted practice. FDA approval of medical devices does not necessarily mean coverage; e.g., if there is a difference between labeled indication and average use (HCFA, 1989-4306-7).

2. HCFA's name was changed to the Centers for Medicare and Medicaid Services (CMS) in 2001.

3. In *Jameson v. Brown*, the plaintiff sued HCFA for reimbursement of a percutaneous transluminal coronary angioplasty conducted before a coverage determination had been made. In addition to reimbursement, HCFA agreed to publish a notice detailing the criteria it used in its coverage process (Federal Register, 1987; Strongin, 2001).

4. Signers of the letter included: the American College of Physicians; American Medical Association; American Society for Internal Medicine; Biotechnology Industry Organization; College of American Pathologists; Council on Radionuclides and Radiopharmaceuticals, Inc.; Health Industry Manufacturers Association; National Electrical Manufacturers Association; and the Pharmaceutical Research and Manufacturers Association of America.

5. A few provisions of the 1989 proposed rule were implemented, such as the treatment of investigational device exemption (IDE)—that certain devices with IDE

and related services will be covered by Medicare for category B, which are certain non-experimental/investigational devices with incremental risks—but where basic issues of safety and efficacy have been established (Federal Register, 1995).

6. Most Medicare coverage decisions are made by local Medicare carriers. In practice, most coverage decisions have been made by Medicare's local contractors— the state or region-wide health insurers (called carriers and fiscal intermediaries), who pay claims for the program. This policy reflects a political compromise to those who wanted to maintain the program's decentralized structure, and a bow to practical considerations, given the dynamic world of medical technology innovation (Foote, 2002; Foote, 2003; Neumann et al., 2004). CMS has noted that it is not always prudent to issue a prescriptive national coverage decision "due to regional, local, or institutional differences in the practice of medicine" (*U.S. Federal Register*, 2000). They stated: "Sometimes there is not sufficient information for us to determine whether an item or service is an effective treatment on a national basis. In other circumstances, there are legitimate regional differences in the practice of medicine that would make a preemptive national rule inappropriate." In addition, only a third of the national coverage decisions that HCFA has issued since MCAC established have gone through MCAC. There is no formal review if evidence is overwhelming in one direction or other (Garber-01).

7. The old mission statement read: "Our essential priority is to provide exceptional quality, cost-effective care strengthened by excellence in education and research." The revised mission statement reads: "To improve human life through excellence in the science and art of health care and healing."

8. The FDA regulates the blood industry through regulations, industry guidance, and memoranda. Normally, a regulatory agency would be required to make a cost estimate for a new regulation under the Regulatory Flexibility Act or section 202(a) of Unfunded Mandates Reform Act. But FDA regulations on blood were issued through *guidance* rather than formal rule-making. The blood industry felt obligated to respond to the guidance because of concerns over legal liability. This complicated the effort for higher Medicare payments, because Medicare couldn't point to formal regulatory cost estimates in order to justify higher payments (O'Grady, 2002).

Chapter 4

1. Thomas says: "Well, the difference between their position and our position is time, and that something that may be more expensive or require a payment at the front end over time, is in fact cost-effective, if you look at the total dollars that would have been spent. What was the mindset in the late eighties, the early nineties or even now in terms of a timeframe reference vis-à-vis what you would call cost-effective. . . . What is the time factor in cost-effectiveness, if any?" Later he says: "Dr. [John] Eisenberg, was there any indication that perhaps a quality-of-life factor could be built into an analysis of a cost-effective [sic] study?" (U.S. Congress, 1997).

2. A similar problem plagues cost-benefit analyses, including those conducted since 1981 for the U.S. government for economically significant federal regulations

under President Reagan's Executive Order 12,291 and President Clinton's Executive Order 12,866. A recent study found that a significant percentage of analyses conducted by the Environmental Protection Agency (EPA) over the past 20 years failed to provide some very basic economic information, such as information on net benefits and policy alternatives. The study found no evidence of improvement over time (Hahn et al., 2000; 2002).

3. Studies show that existing analyses are very inconsistent in the source of preferences, and most often authors simply use their own judgments rather than preferences from patient or community samples (Neumann et al., 1997; Bell et al., 2000).

4. It is not clear, however, whether these kinds of differences in preference weights change ultimate study conclusions. A recent paper investigating the impact of quality-of-life adjustment on cost-effectiveness analyses found that in a sizable fraction of cost-utility analyses, quality adjusting did not substantially alter the estimated cost-effectiveness of an intervention, suggesting that sensitivity analyses using ad hoc adjustments or "off-the-shelf" utility weights may be sufficient for many analyses (Chapman et al., in press).

5. Cost-utility analysis has its roots in expected utility theory (von-Neumann Morgenstern), which describes a normative model of rational decision-making under conditions of uncertainty. The preference or quality weights that are developed from preferences developed with methods other than the standard gamble are thus not technically utilities. But even QALYs developed with preferences constructed from standard gambles are only utilities if several restrictive assumptions hold. These conditions include *independence of preferences* (utility scales for length of life and quality of life can be specified independently rather than conditionally upon the level of the other attribute); *constant proportional tradeoffs* between longevity and quality of life (one would be willing to give up some fraction of one's life years in order to improve the quality of those years from one level to a preferred level, and that the fraction depends only on the two quality levels and not on the length of life at the outset; and *risk neutrality* (utilities are directly proportional to longevity for a fixed quality level) (Weinstein and Fineberg, 1980; Drummond et al., 1997). QALYs can be represented by a more general, risk-adjusted model if the utility independence and constant proportional tradeoff assumptions hold (Pliskin et al., 1980). To date, only a few studies have examined the empirical evidence for the descriptive validity of QALYs as utilities, with mixed results reported (Bleichrodt and Johannesson, 1996; Bryan et al., 2002).

6. Countries using mandatory or voluntary guidelines include Australia, Canada, Finland, the Netherlands, Denmark, Ireland, New Zealand, Norway, Switzerland, and the United Kingdom (Hjelmgren et al., 2001).

7. In one recent study of 228 cost-utility analyses published between 1976 and 1997, only 23% of the ratios were above $50,000 per QALY, for example, and only 13% over $100,000 per QALY. Of the 76 ratios above $100,000, only 3 (4%) were industry-sponsored (Neumann et al., 2000b).

8. Neumann et al. (2000b) reported that of 228 cost-utility analyses published between 1976 and 1997, industry-funded studies actually fared slightly better than

those funded by non-industry sources on an overall quality score, though the difference was not statistically significant. Also, investigators of industry-sponsored studies were much more likely to disclose their source of funding (which could simply reflect journals' disclosure requirements regarding industry funding. But the investigators did not test the quality of the actual clinical and economic assumptions made in analyses, only whether recommended protocols were followed.

Chapter 5

1. The draft guidelines noted that "models to provide estimates of pharmacoeconomic parameters should be used only when it is impractical or impossible to gather data using adequate and well-controlled trials" (U.S. FDA, 1995).

2. This section is adapted in part from Neumann et al., 2000c.

3. For example, in conceptualizing medical necessity, some have distinguished a treatment/enhancement paradigm—services to prevent, cure, or ameliorate impairment are distinguished from those that merely improve conditions that are part of normal human functioning (Daniels and Sabin, 1994, cited in Studdert and Gresenz, 2002). But "cost-effectiveness" has not been part of the conception.

4. To date, however, courts do not appear to have used CEA when instructing juries (Jacobson and Kanna, 2001).

5. In *Pegram v. Herdrich*, 2000, in which the U.S. Supreme Court ruled unanimously in favor of a physician who made decisions that entailed slightly higher risks but reduced costs, Justice Souter stated: "Imposing federal liability for efforts to reduce costs—the entire purpose of managed care—could destroy HMOs altogether. . . ." He added that: "inducement to ration care goes to the very point of any HMO scheme and rationing necessarily raises some risks while reducing others" (cited in Eddy, 2001).

6. Most of the regulatory impact analyses submitted in response to EO 12,866 have addressed environmental and occupational safety regulations rather than health (e.g., Medicare) regulations per se. Similarly, while some federal statutes over the years have also included mandates to balance costs and benefits, or to consider risk-risk tradeoffs, or evaluate the cost-effectiveness of different regulatory alternatives, they have generally pertained to environmental regulations (e.g., the Safe Drinking Water Act Amendments of 1996, the Small Business Enforcement and Fairness Act of 1996; and the Unfunded Mandates Reform Act of 1995 [Hahn, 2000]).

7. In a study of 228 CUAs published between 1976 and 1997, 78 (34%) of the articles mention an explicit dollar threshold for this value, with a median amount of $50,000 (Neumann et al., 2000b).

8. A sizeable body of work has arisen over the years on this issue. It is beyond the scope of this book to critique all of these studies—good recent summaries are provided in Nord (1999); Ubel (2000); and Daniels and Sabin (2002).

9. The Panel notes that incorporating preference subgroups may not be feasible for purposes of the Reference Case, but if important, they should be highlighted in the discussion section (Gold et al., 1996, p. 103).

Chapter 6

1. The Medicaid Program provides medical assistance for certain individuals and families with low incomes and resources. Medicaid eligibility is limited to individuals who fall into specific categories, which depend on the state in which he or she lives, though the rules are subject to general federal guidelines for the program (www.cms.gov).

2. Because the Oregon plan amended the basic Medicaid program, the state was required to obtain a waiver from the federal Health Care Financing Administration under demonstration authority conferred by Section 1115 of the Social Security Act. While the state might have pursued a congressional fix (i.e., getting Congress to pass legislation giving Oregon the authority), it followed the federal option instead (Fox and Leichter, 1993).

3. The plan retained some of the other original features, such as covering residents up to 100% of the poverty line, simplifying rules for participating in the program so that eligibility was based only on income, encouraging managed-care delivery, and securing higher reimbursement for managed-care delivery (Fox, Leicter, 1993). The original employer mandate for health insurance lapsed over a failure to obtain a federal waiver (Ham, 1998).

4. Some have disputed Oregon's claims about the decline of its uninsured population (e.g., Himmelstein and Woolhandler, 1998).

5. As one example, in 1995 the legislature modified the eligibility criteria so that an eligible individual's average income must be below the poverty line for three months instead of one month. In addition, eligibility for students was eliminated (Kilborn, 1999). On the other hand, the state has also expanded coverage to other populations over the years (e.g., pregnant women with incomes up to 150% of the federal poverty line [Leichter, 1999]).

6. In 1997, the legislature wanted to move from the line from 581 to 574 but HCFA only allowed a move to 578 (Bodenheim, 1997).

7. Other countries have found ways to prioritize resources more explicitly, as discussed in chapter 8.

8. The employer mandate would have required the state to receive an exemption from Congress from the Employee Retirement Income Security Act (ERISA), which was never a possibility in the Republican-controlled Congress of the mid-1990s (Leichter, 1999).

9. A new waiver for Oregon was approved in October 2002, which would allow in effect [two benefits—OHP Plus,] which is the existing benefit package for categorically eligible, plus OHP Standard, for others not categorically eligible.

Chapter 7

1. The Health Economics Evaluation Database lists 3,116 original CEAs (i.e., excluding methods or review papers) published between 1975 through 2000 (533 cost/LY analyses, 512 cost/QALY analyses, and 2,071 CEAs using other metrics

[e.g., cost per cancer case prevented]). The database also lists 97 original cost-benefit analyses published during the same period (author's calculation from OHE database).

2. A comprehensive list of cost-utility analyses published through 2001 is available at www.hsph.harvard.edu/cearegistry.

3. Medicare has added preventative services on other occasions. Most notably, the Balanced Budget Act of 1997 included or expanded coverage for diabetes management, screening for osteoporosis, and screening for prostate, colorectal, cervical, and breast cancer. But generally services were added in an ad hoc fashion, not subject in a formal or consistent manner to cost-effectiveness analysis, and in some cases not even consistent with U.S. Task Force on Clinical Prevention recommendations (MedPAC, 2002).

4. The Notice comments that *substantially more beneficial* could be construed to be whether physicians believe the new technology defines a new standard. The Notice also states that "although mortality and life-expectancy are quantifiable and thus 'hard' health outcomes, we believe that we should move towards 'quality of life' as an acceptable health outcome . . . we seek suggestions on quality adjusted life years. . . ."

The Notice also solicits input on the terms *same clinical modality* and *Medicare-covered alternative*.

5. The Balanced Budget Refinement Act (BBRA) of 1999 established pass-through payments for certain types of new technology for the outpatient prospective payment system, and the Medicare, Medicaid, and SCHIP Benefits Improvement and Protection Act (BIPA) of 2000 requires CMS to develop new mechanisms to pay for technological advances under inpatient PPS.

6. As of September 2003, the states included Florida, Idaho, Indiana, Louisiana, Oregon, Washington, Utah, Michigan, Mississippi, and Alabama.

7. This section is adopted in part from Neumann PJ, Evidence-based and value-based formulary guidelines, *Health Affairs*, 2004.

8. The strategies were: bicycle-related head injuries, breast cancer, cervical cancer, childhood lead poisoning, childhood vaccine-preventable diseases, chlamydia-related infertility, colorectal cancer, coronary heart disease, dental caries, diabetic retinopathy, HIV/AIDS transmission, influenza among elderly persons, low birthweight, neural tube defects, perinatal hepatitis B, pneumococcal disease, sickle cell screening in newborns, smoking, and tuberculosis (CDC, 1999).

9. Executive Order 12,866 states

> In deciding whether and how to regulate, agencies should assess all costs and benefits of available regulatory alternatives, including the alternative of not regulating. Costs and benefits shall be understood to include both quantifiable measures (to the fullest extent that these can be usefully estimated) and qualitative measures of costs and benefits that are difficult to quantify, but nevertheless essential to consider. Further, in choosing among alternative regulatory approaches, agencies should select those approaches that maximize net benefits (including potential economic, environmental, public health and safety, and other advantages; distributive impacts; and

equity), unless a statute requires another regulatory approach. (5) When an agency determines that a regulation is the best available method of achieving the regulatory objective, it shall design its regulations in the most cost-effective manner to achieve the regulatory objective. In doing so, each agency shall consider incentives for innovation, consistency, predictability, the costs of enforcement and compliance (to the government, regulated entities, and the public), flexibility, distributive impacts, and equity. (6) Each agency shall assess both the costs and the benefits of the intended regulation and, recognizing that some costs and benefits are difficult to quantify, propose or adopt a regulation only upon a reasoned determination that the benefits of the intended regulation justify its costs. (7) Each agency shall base its decisions on the best reasonably obtainable scientific, technical, economic, and other information concerning the need for, and consequences of, the intended regulation.

Note that OMB only reviews rulemaking issued by executive agencies, not independent agencies. Of about 4,500 federal rulemakings each year, 600 are significant enough to justify OMB review, and 50–100 are considered "major" or "economically significant" (OBM, 2003).

10. The report, which is subject to a 60-day public comment period and expert peer review, is required by the Regulatory Right to Know Act of 2000, requiring OMB to update periodically its guidelines for regulatory analysis (OMB, 2003). The 2003 report updates OMB best practices guidelines from 1996.

Chapter 8

1. In 2002, the Australian Pharmaceutical Benefits Scheme (PBS) covered more than 620 drugs, more than 230 of which (37%) had been included following explicit cost-effectiveness considerations (Mitchell, 2002). Drugs must first be approved for marketing by the Therapeutic Goods Administration (TGA), which considers safety, efficacy, and quality, but not cost or cost-effectiveness. Drugs approved for the market may also be purchased privately.

2. Enforcement is not perfect—partly due to pharmaceutical marketing, which can influence use outside of the restricted area, an area of controversy currently being pursued in the Australian courts. Theoretically, there could be different prices in and out of restriction, or a price could be weighted by two indications if the drug has a competitor for one indication and not the other (Mitchell, personal communication, August 2002).

3. Lipman (2001) wrote that NICE is the kind of "centralized, bureaucratic system that has hamstrung the NHS for decades . . . [and that its] traditional panoply of expert committees and top-down implementation guidelines have claimed legitimacy by invoking the mantra of evidence-based medicine."

4. The NICE chairman, Michael Rawlins, stated that the notion of a threshold beyond which rejection is automatic is an "urban myth," but observers pointed to use of the word "automatic" in this utterance as proof that a threshold, in fact, exists (Towse and Pritchard, 2002).

Chapter 10

1. This section is adapted in part from Neumann et al., 2000d.

2. In recent years, for example, researchers have experimented with various alternative elicitation techniques, including estimating general-population utilities using one binary-gamble question per respondent (Bosch et al., 1998), and using "chained procedures" to measure temporary health states (temporary health states weighed indirectly with the aid of intermediate anchor states) (Janset et al., 1998). Methods for optimizing sampling strategies for estimating QALYs have also been explored (Ramsey et al., 1997). The elicitation protocol used to search for subjects' utility values can strongly influence results (Lenert et al., 1998), but telephone interviews yield similar time–tradeoff values and standard gamble utilities compared to face-to-face interviews (Van Wijck et al., 1998).

3. There is already some precedent for this: Executive Order 12,866 requires that qualitative description of equity be presented to regulators in the rulemaking process (U.S. Office of Management and Budget, 2002).

4. Healthy-years equivalents (HYEs) have been proposed as an alternative to QALYs (Gafni and Birch, 1993, Mehrez and Gafni, 1989; Mehrez and Gafni, 1993) on the basis that they avoid certain restrictive assumptions about preferences. For example, supporters claim that HYEs generalize from constant proportionality of QALYs by permitting the rate of tradeoff between life years and quality of life to depend on the lifespan. HYEs are calculated by measuring the utility for each possible "health pathway" of a stream of changing health states and converting this utility to an HYE by a second measurement. There is, however, considerable debate about this second component, which has been shown to be essentially equivalent to a simple time-tradeoff question (Wakker, 1996; Morrison, 1997). Johannesson et al. (1993) argue that HYEs are by definition the same as the equivalent number of years in full health in the time tradeoff developed by Torrance et al. (1972)—that they are essentially a generalization of risk-neutral QALYs in which the assumption of a constant proportional tradeoff between life years and quality of life is relaxed. Furthermore, the difficulty of utility assessment is appreciable because the number of HYEs must be calculated for every possible duration of time in the health state. In other words, they require independent valuations of all possible health scenarios rather than individual health states (Johannesson et al., 1993). Thus, HYEs do not offer a practical solution to the problem of assigning utilities to health profiles for varying qualities of life because of the enormous scope of the task of assessing time tradeoffs for all possible sequences of health states over a lifetime.

Disability-adjusted life years (DALY) have been widely used in economic evaluations conducted outside the United States (Murray and Lopez, 1996), and in many international health interventions report health outcomes as cost per DALY have been defined (Jamieson et al., 1996). DALYs were developed as the measurement unit for the Global Burden of Disease Study (Murray and Lopez, 1996), whose goal was to quantify the burden of disease and injury in human populations. In effect, DALYs are similar to QALYs in that they provide a metric for quantifying life expectancy after adjusting for morbidity. Where QALY weights are based on social preferences, however, DALY weights also incorporate age adjustments, based implicitly on economic productivity (i.e., young or middle-aged adults receive higher weights than the elderly or small children). DALYs are not without their own critics. Some have raised questions about the equity and ethics of the age-weightings, for example (Morrow et al., 1995). Also, DALYs rely on Japanese life tables no matter what the actual target population.

5. Where some studies have suggested that the problem of poor reporting practice is particularly acute in clinical specialty journals (Udhvarhelyi et al., 1992; Gerard et al., 1999), more recent analysis implicates a journal's inexperience in publishing cost-utility analyses, rather than the type of journal per se (Neumann et al., 2000). In a regression analysis predicting overall subjective quality score as a function of journal type and volume, volume was a positive and significant predictor (p = .024), whereas the type of journal was not significant.

Chapter 11

1. Jacobson and Kanna (2001) point out that in the 1974 *Helling v. Carey* case in which women under 40 were not screened for glaucoma, the court said "low cost relative to benefit" was a reason for overriding professional custom, though they note that most courts reject Helling, relying on professional custom model.

Hall v. Hilbun, 1985, examined the question of whether local or national standards should prevail. The courts said that the duty of care should be based on the adept use of facilities, services reasonably available (e.g., a rural hospital might have less). Jacobson and Kanna (2001) note that this could be expanded to incorporate CEA or CBA—retain professional standards but permit the profession to factor in resource constraints.

2. In its 2000 Notice on criteria for coverage, for example, CMS acknowledged that they needed input on when a service would constitute the "same clinical modality" and what would be "substantially more beneficial"—for example, whether physicians believe it defines a new standard (*U.S. Federal Register*, 2000).

3. As far as what constitutes this evidence, she notes that HCFA will rely on controlled clinical trials, controlled studies, or case studies; formal technology assessments from recognized government and private entities, which examine published and unpublished data; evaluations from Medicare contractors; and authoritative approvals from other agencies, e.g., FDA (DeParle, 1998). Later, CMS, in developing MCAC criteria on the adequacy of evidence, notes that the validity of the evidence and its general applicability to the population of interest . . . "many forms of evidence can be valid or not, depending on the circumstances, and will depend on factors, such as bias; external validity; size of health effect—breakthrough technology, more effective, as effective but with advantages, as effective with no advantages; less effective but with advantages; less effective and with no advantages; not effective; and the possibility of developing evidence—e.g., the cost of performing the study is high and funding has not been available" (HCFA, 2000).

4. CMS, in proposing its criteria for making its coverage process more open, responsive, and understandable, recognized this, stating that "we anticipate that the criteria would result in covering more items and services under Medicare. . . ." (*U.S. Federal Register*, 2000).

5. Publicity about financial incentives were only published as a result of a lawsuit settlement (Freudenheim, 2003).

References

Aaron HJ, Schwartz WB. *The painful prescription*. The Brookings Institution: Washington, DC, 1984.

Acton JP. *Evaluating public programs to save lives: The case of heart attacks*. R-950-RC. Rand: Santa Monica, CA, 1973.

Adam T, Evans DB, Koopmanschap. Cost-effectiveness analysis: Can we reduce variability in costing methods? *International Journal of Technology Assessment in Health Care* 2003;19(2):407–420.

Adams ME, McCall NT, Gray DT, Orza MJ, Chalmers TC. Economic analysis in randomized controlled trials. *Medical Care* 1992:30:231–238.

Agency for Health Care Research and Quality. MEPS HC-020: 1997 Full Year Consolidated Data File. Available at www.meps.ahrq.gov/Puf/PufDetail.asp?ID=36. Accessed March 21, 2003.

Agency for Health Care Research and Quality. Home page, www.ahrq.gov. Accessed September 17, 2003.

Agency for Health Care Research and Quality. Focus on Cost-Effectiveness Analysis at AHRQ. Available at www.ahcpr.gov/research/costeff.htm. Accessed on October 2, 2003.

Akehurst R. The influence of economic evaluation in the health care environment: Some reflections. In JL Pinto, G Lopez-Casasnovas, and V Ortun (eds). *Economic evaluation: From theory to practice*. Springer-Verlag Iberica: Barcelona, 2001, pp. 163–178.

Akehurst R. Drug evaluation process: The U.K. and European models. Presentation at the 14th Annual Meeting of the Academy of Managed Care Pharmacy. Salt Lake City, Utah, April 5, 2002.

AMCP News. "AMCP Approves Drafting of Guidelines for Formulary Submissions." Academy of Managed Care Pharmacy: Alexandria, VA, July 1998.

AMCP Format for Formulary Submissions. Academy of Managed Care Pharmacy, Alexandria, VA. Version 2.0. (October 2002). Available at: http://www.amcp.org/publications/format.pdf. Accessed on February 5, 2003.

American College of Physicians, et al. Letter to Bruce Vladeck, Administrator of the Health Care Financing Administration. September 23, 1996.

Anand G. The big secret in health care: Rationing is here. *Wall Street Journal*, September 12, 2003, p. A1.

Anderson GF, Hall MA, Steinberg EP. Medical technology assessment and practice guidelines: Their day in court. *American Journal of Public Health* 1993;83: 1635–39.

Anderson GF, Hall MA, Smith TR. When courts review medical appropriateness. *Medical Care* 1998;36(8):1295–1302.

Anell A, Svarvar P. Pharmacoeconomic and clinical practice guidelines: A survey of attitudes in Swedish formulary committees. *Pharmacoeconomics* 2000:17(2):175–185.

Anis AH, Gagnon Y. Using economic evaluations to make formulary coverage decisions: So much for guidelines. *Pharmacoeconomics* 2000;18(1):55–62.

Arrow KJ. Uncertainty and the welfare economics of medical care. *American Economic Review* 1963;53:941–973.

Arrow KJ. Behavior under uncertainty and its implications for policy. In Bell DE, Raiffa H, Tversky A, eds. *Decision making: Descriptive, normative, and prescriptive interactions*. Cambridge University Press: New York, 1988, pp. 497–507.

Asch DA, Ubel PA. Rationing by any other name. *New England Journal of Medicine* 1997;336:1668–1671.

Asch DA, Jepson C, Hershey JC, Baron J, Ubel PA. When money is saved by reducing health care costs, where do U.S. physicians think the money goes? *American Journal of Managed Care* 2003 Jun;9(6):438–42.

Atherly DE, Sullivan SD, Fullerton DS, Sturm LL. Incorporating clinical outcomes and economic consequences into drug formulary decisions: Evaluation of 30 months of experience. *Value in Health* [abstract] 2001;4(2):52.

AuBuchon JP. Cost-effectiveness of new blood safety technologies. *Developing Biological Standards* 2000;102:211–215.

Ayanian J, Cleary JD. Perceived risks of heart disease and cancer among cigarette smokers. *Journal of the American Medical Association* 1999;281:1019–1021.

Azimi NA, Welch HG. The effectiveness of cost-effectiveness analysis in containing costs. *Journal of General Internal Medicine* 1998;13:664–669.

Balaban DJ, Sagi PC, Goldfarb NI, Nettler S. Weights for scoring the quality of well-being instrument among rheumatoid athritics: A comparison to general population weights. *Medical Care* 1986;24:973–80.

Balas EA, Kretschmer RAC, Gnann W, et al. Interpreting cost analyses of clinical interventions. *Journal of the American Medical Association* 1998;279:54–57.

Begg CB. "Publication bias." In H. Cooper and L.V. Hedges, eds, *The handbook of research synthesis*. Russell Sage Foundation: New York, 1994.

Bell CM, Chapman RH, Stone PW, Sandberg EA, and Neumann PJ. An off-the-shelf help list: A comprehensive catalogue of preference scores from published cost-utility analyses. *Medical Decision Making* 2001;21:288–94.

Berger ML. The once and future application of cost-effectiveness analysis. *Journal of Quality Improvement* 1999;25(9):455–461.

Birch S, Gafni A. Cost-effectiveness ratios: In a league of their own. *Health Policy* 1994;28:133–141.

Blackmore CC, Magid DJ. Methodologic evaluation of the radiology cost-effectiveness literature. *Radiology* 1997;203:87–91.

Bleichrodt H, Johannesson M. An experimental test of constant proportional tradeoff and utility independence. *Medical Decision Making* 1996;17:21–32.

Bleichrodt H, Johannesson M. An experimental test of the theoretical foundation for rating scale valuations. *Medical Decision Making* 1997;17(2):208–216.

Blendon RJ, Leitman R, Morrison I, Donelan K. Satisfaction with health systems in ten nations. *Health Affairs* 1990;9(2):185–192.

Blendon RJ, Brodie M, Benson JM, Altman DE, Levitt L, Hoff T, Hugick L. Understanding the managed care backlash. *Health Affairs* 1998;17(4):80–94.

Blue Cross Blue Shield of Colorado, Blue Cross Blue Shield of Nevada. Guidelines for Formulary Submissions for Pharmaceutical Product Evaluation. Denver, Colorado. October 1998.

Blumenthal D. Federal Policy toward health care technology: The case of the National Center. Milbank Memorial Fund Quarterly Health Society 1983;61(4): 584–613.

Blumenthal D, Gluck M, Louis KS., Stoto MA, Wise D. University-industry research relationships in biotechnology: Implications for the university. *Science* 232 (1986): 1361–1366.

Bodenheimer T. The Oregon health plan—Lessons for the nation. *New England Journal of Medicine* 1997;337(9):651–655.

Bogardus et al. Perils, pitfalls, and possibilities in talking about medical risk. *Journal of the American Medical Association* 1999;281:1037–1041.

Bombardier C, Ware J, Russell IJ, Larson M, Chalmers A, Read JL. Auranofin therapy and quality of life in patients with rheumatoid arthritis: Results of a multicenter trial. *American Journal of Medicine* 1986;81:565–581.

Bosch JL, Hunink MGM, Tetteroo E, Bos JJ, Mali WPThM. 1994. Quality of life assessment in patients with peripheral arterial disease. *Medical Decision Making* 14(4):425 (abstract).

Bosch JL, Hunink MGM. 1996. The relationship between descriptive and valuational quality-of-life measures in patients with intermittent claudication. *Medical Decision Making* 165:217–225.

Bosch JL, Hammitt JK, Weinstein JC, and Hunink MGM. 1998. Estimating general population utilities using one binary-gamble question per respondent. *Medical Decision Making* 18:381–390.

Bottorff JL, Ratner PA, Johnson JL, et al. Communicating cancer risk information: The challenges of uncertainty. *Patient Education Counseling* 1998;33:67–81.

Box GEP, Hunter WG, Hunter JS. Statistics for experimenters: An introduction to design, data analysis, and model building. John Wiley & Sons: New York, 1978.

Brazier J, Jones N, Kind P. A comparison of two health status measures: Euroqol meets SF-36. Presentation at the Health Economics Study Group/Faculty of Public Health Medicine Conference, University of York, York, U.K., January, 1993.

Briggs AH, Sculpher M. Sensitivity analysis in economic evaluation: A review of published studies. *Health Economics* 1995;4:355–371.

Briggs AH, Wonderling DE, Mooney CZ. Pulling cost-effectiveness analysis up by its bootstraps: A nonparametric approach to confidence interval estimation. *Health Economics* 1997;6(4):327–340.

Briggs AH, O'Brien BJ, Blackhouse G. Thinking outside the box: Recent advances in the analysis and presentation of uncertainty in cost-effectiveness studies. *Annual Review of Public Health* 2002;23:377–401.

Brown LD. The national politics of Oregon's rationing plan. *Health Affairs* 1991; 10(2):28–51.

Brown ML, Fintor L. Cost-effectiveness of breast cancer screening: preliminary results of a systematic review of the literature. *Breast Cancer Research and Treatment* 1993; 25:113–118.

Brouwer WBF, Koopmanschap MA, Rutten FFH. Patient and informal caregiver time in cost-effectiveness analysis: A response to the recommendations of the Washington Panel. *International Journal of Technology Assessment in Health Care* 1998;14:505–513.

Burke K. No cash to implement NICE, health authorities tell MPs. *British Medical Journal* 2002;324:258.

Buto K. How can Medicare keep pace with cutting-edge technology? *Health Affairs* 1994;13(3):137–140.

Campen D. The bleeding edge of decision making in managed health care—Kaiser Permanente's model for formulary development. *Value in Health* 2002;5(5): 383–89.

Canadian Coordinating Office for Health Technology Assessment. Available at http://www.ccohta.ca/entry_e.html. Accessed September 18, 2003.

Carande-Kulis VG, Maciosek MV, Briss PA, et al. Methods for systematic reviews of economic evaluations for the Guide to Community Preventive Services. *American Journal of Preventive Medicine* 2000;18(1S):75–91.

Carrasquillo O, Lantigua RA, Shea S. Preventive services among Medicare beneficiaries with supplemental coverage versus HMO enrollees, Medicaid recipients and elders with no additional coverage. *Medical Care* 2001;39(6):616–626.

Centers for Disease Control and Prevention. An ounce of prevention: What are the returns? CDC's Prevention Effectiveness Branch, Division of Prevention Research and Analytic Methods: Atlanta, GA, 1999.

Center for Studying Health System Change. "Issue Brief: Wall Street comes to Washington." July 2002.

Chapman RH, Stone PW, Sandberg EA, Bell C, Neumann PJ. A comprehensive league table of cost-utility ratios and a sub-table of "Panel-worthy" studies. *Medical Decision Making* 2000;20:451–467.

Chapman RH, Berger ML, Weinstein MC, Weeks JC, Goldie SJ, Neumann PJ. *When Do Quality-Adjusting Life-Years matter in cost-effectiveness Analysis?* Health Economics. In press. 2002.

Chapman S, Reeve E, Rajaratnam G, Neary R. Setting up an outcomes guarantee for pharmaceuticals: New approach to risk sharing in primary care. *British Medical Journal* 2003;326:707–709.

Cheap cures. Donors should give more, but the poor should spend what they have more rationally. *The Economist.* August 17, 2002, pp. 13–14.

Claxton K, Posnett J. An economic approach to clinical trial design and research priority setting. *Health Economics* 1996;5(6):513–524.

Claxton K. The irrelevance of inference: A decision-making approach to the stochastic evaluation of health care technologies. *Journal of Health Economics* 1999;18(3):341–364.

Claxton K, Neumann PJ, Araki S, Weinstein MC. Bayesian value-of-information analysis: An application to a policy model of Alzheimer's disease. *International Journal of Technology Assessment in Health Care* 2001;17(1):38–55.

Clemens K, Garrison L, Jones A, Macdonald F. Strategic use of pharmacoeconomic research in early drug development and global pricing. *Pharmacoeconomics* 1993;4(5):315–322.

Cohen J, Krauss N. Spending and service use among people with the fifteen most costly medical conditions, 1997. *Health Affairs* 2003;22(2):129–138.

Cookson R. ASTEC Non-EU case study on Australia. London School of Economics and Political Science: July 2000.

Corso PS, Thacker SB, Koplan JP. The value of prevention: Experiences of a public health agency. *Medical Decision Making* 2002;22(Suppl):S11–16.

Cross MA. Formulary submission process catches on . . . slowly. *Managed Care* November 2002:32–36.

Crump B, Drummond MF, Alexander S, Devaney C. Economic evaluation in the United Kingdom National Health Service. In Schulenburg J-M Graf v d, ed. *The influence of economic evaluation studies on health care decision making: A European survey*. IOS Press: Amsterdam, 2000.

Daniels N. Is the Oregon rationing plan fair? *Journal of the American Medical Association* 1991;265:2232–2235.

Daniels N. Four unsolved rationing problems. *Hastings Center Report* 1994;24(4):27–29.

Daniels N, Sabin JE. Determining "medical necessity" in mental health practices: A study of clinical reasoning and a proposal for insurance policy. *Hastings Center Report* 1994;22(6):5–13.

Daniels N, Sabin JE. *Setting limits fairly*. Oxford University Press: New York, 2002.

Daniels N, Teagarden JR, Sabin JE. An ethical template for pharmacy benefits. *Health Affairs* 2003;22(1):125–137.

Darba J, Rovira J, Papadopoulus T. The transferability of results of economic evaluation studies. In Pinto JL, Lopez-Casasnovas G, and Ortun V, eds. *Economic evaluation: From theory to practice*. Springer-Verlag Iberica: Barcelona, 2001, pp. 119–128.

Dent THS, Sadler M. From guidance to practice: Why NICE is not enough. *British Medical Journal* 2002;324:842–845.

Detsky A. Are clinical trials a cost-effective investment? *Journal of the American Medical Association* 1989;262:1795–1800.

Detsky AS. Using cost-effectiveness analysis for formulary decision making. *Pharmacoeconomics* 1994;6(4):281–288.

Devlin N. Cost-effectiveness thresholds in decision making: What are the issues? In A Towse, C Pritchard, N Devlin, eds. *Cost-effectiveness thresholds, economic and ethical issues*. OHE: London, 2002.

Deyo RA, Psaty BM, Simon G, Wagner EH, Omenn GS. The messenger under attack—Intimidation of researchers by special-interest groups. *New England Journal of Medicine* 1997;336(16):1176–80.

Dillon MJ. Drug formulary management. In Navarro RP, Ed. *Managed care pharmacy practice* Aspen Publication: Gaithersburg, MD, 1999, pp. 145–166.

DiMasi JA, Caglarcan E, Wood-Armany M. Emerging role of pharmacoeconomics in the research and development decision-making process. *Pharmacoeconomics* 2001;19(7):753–66.

Dolan P. The measurement of individual utility and social welfare. *Health Econonomics* 1998;17:39–52.

Doubilet P, Weinstein MC, McNeil BJ. Use and misuse of the term "cost-effective" in medicine. *New England Journal of Medicine* 1986;314:253–55.

Dranove D. Measuring costs. In Sloan F, ed. *Valuing health care: Costs, benefits, and effectiveness of pharmceuticals and other medical technologies*. Cambridge: Cambridge University Press, 1995.

Drummond MF, Stoddart GL. Economic analysis and clinical trials. *Controlled Clinical Trials* 1984;5(2):115–128.

Drummond MF, Stoddart GL, Torrance GW. *Methods for the Economic Evaluation of Health Care Programmes.* Oxford University Press: Oxford, 1987.

Drummond MF, Jefferson TO (for the Economic Evaluation Workshop Party). Guidelines for authors and peer reviewers of economic submissions to *BMJ*. *British Medical Journal* 1996;313:275–283.

Drummond MF, O'Brien B, Stoddart GL, Torrance GW. *Methods for the Economic Evaluation of Health Care Programmes.* Oxford University Press: Oxford, 1997.

Drummond M, Cooke J, Walley T. Economic evaluation under managed competition: Evidence from the U.K. *Social Science & Medicine* 1997b;45(4):583–95.

Drummond MF, Richardson WS, O'Brien BJ, Levine M, Heyland D (for the Evidence-Based Medicine Working Group). Users' guides to the medical literature: XIII. How to use an article on economic analysis: A. Are the results of the study valid? *Journal of the American Medical Association* 1997c;277;1552–1557.

Drummond M. Current trends in the use of pharmacoeconomics and outcomes research in Europe. *Value in Health* 1999;2:323–332.

Drummond M. Validity of economic evaluations: Obstacles to its use. In Pinto JL, Lopez-Casasnovas G, and Ortun V, eds. *Economic evaluation: From theory to practice.* Springer-Verlag Iberica: Barcelona, 2001:99–112.

Drummond M, McGuire A. *Economic evaluation in health care: Merging theory with practice.* Oxford University Press: Oxford, 2002.

Drummond MF, et al. ISPOR task force on the use of pharmacoeconomic/health economic information in health care decision-making. *ISPOR*, 2002.

Drummond MF and Sculpher M. Common methodological flaws in economic evaluation: Working paper. Centre for Health Economics. York University. 2003. Available at http://www.york.ac.uk/inst/che/public.htm. Accessed September 16, 2003.

Dupuit J. De le mesure de l'utilité des traveaux publics. *Annales de ponts des Chaussées.* Deuxième Série. 1844;8.

Duthie T, Trueman P, Chancellor J, Diez L. Research into the use of health economics in decision making in the United Kingdom—Phase II: Is health economics for good or evil? *Health Policy* 1999;46:143–57.

Earle CC, Chapman RH, Baker CS, Bell CM, Stone PW, Sandberg EA, and Neumann PJ. A systematic overview of cost-utility assessments in oncology. *Journal of Clinical Oncology* 2000;18:3302–3317.

Eckstein O. *Water resource development: The economics of project evaluation.* Harvard University Press: Cambridge, MA, 1958.

Eddy DM. Screening for breast cancer. *Annals of Internal Medicine* 1989;111:389–399.

——. Screening for colorectal cancer. *Annals of Internal Medicine* 1990a;113:373–384.

——. Screening for cervical cancer. *Annals of Internal Medicine* 1990b;113:214–226.

——. Oregon's methods: Did cost-effectiveness fail? *Journal of the American Medical Association* 1991;266:2135–2141.

——. Cost-effectiveness analysis: A conversation with my father. *Journal of the American Medical Association* 1992a;267:1669–1675.

——. Applying cost-effectiveness analysis: The inside story. *Journal of the American Medical Association* 1992b;268:2575–2582.

——. Cost-effectiveness analysis: Is it up to the task? *Journal of the American Medical Association* 1992c;267:3342–3348.

——. Cost-effectiveness analysis: Will it be accepted? *Journal of the American Medical Association* 1992d;268:132–36.

——. Benefit language: Criteria that will improve quality while reducing costs. *Journal of the American Medical Association* 1996;275:650–57.

——. Performance measurement: Problems and solutions. *Health Affairs* 1998;17:7–25.

——. The use of evidence and cost-effectiveness by the courts: How can it help improve health care? *Journal of Health Politics, Policy and Law* 2001;26(2): 387–408.

Elixhauser A, Luce BR, Taylor WR, Reblando J. Health care CBA/CEA: An update on the growth and composition of the literature. *Medical Care* 1993;31:JS1–JS138.

Elixhauser A, Halpern M, Schmier J, and Luce BR. Health care CBA and CEA from 1991 to 1996: An updated bibliography. *Medical Care* 1998;36:MS1–MS9.

Ellis. Doctors treating patients with multiple sclerosis will lose confidence in NICE. Letter to editor, *British Medical Journal* 2001;322:489.

Elstein A. *MDM* policy regarding financial support of authors. *Medical Decision Making* 1997;17:497–498.

Epstein AM, Hall JA, Tognetti J., et al. 1989. Using proxies to evaluate quality of life: Can they provide valid information about patients' health status and satisfaction with medical care? *Medical Care* 27(suppl):S91–98.

Etzioni RD, Feuer EJ, Sullivan SD, Lin D, Hu C, Ramsey SD. On the use of survival analysis techniques to estimate medical costs. *Journal of Health Economics* 1999:18(3):365–380.

Evans R. Manufacturing consensus, marketing truth: Guidelines for economic evaluation. *Annals of Internal Medicine* 1995;123:59–60.

Evans C, Dukes EM, Crawford B. The role of pharmacoeconomic information in the Formulary decision-making process. *Journal of Managed Care Pharmacy.* 2000;6(2):113–121.

EuroQol Group. 1990. EuroQol–a new facility for the measurement of health related quality of life. *Health Policy* 16:199–208.

Fang CC, Hay J, Wallace JF, Bloom B., Neumann PJ, Sullivan SD, Yu HT, Keeler AB, Henning JM, Ofman JJ. Development and validation of a grading system for the quality of cost-effectiveness studies. *Medical Care* 2003;41:32–44.

Feeny DH and Torrance GW. Incorporating utility-based quality-of-life assessment measures in a randomised trial. *Medical Care* 1989;27(suppl 3):S190–S204.

Feeny D, Furlong W, Torrance GW, Goldsmith CH, Zhu Z, DePauw S, Denton M, Boyle M. Multiattribute and single-attribute utility functions for the health utilities index mark 3 system. *Medical Care* 2002;40(2):113–128.

Fenwick E. *Health technology assessment: The need for an iterative framework.* Centre for Health Economics, University of York: York, U.K., 2003.

Ferguson JH, Dubinsky M, and Kirsch. Court-ordered reimbursement for unproven medical technology: Circumventing technology assessment. *Journal of the American Medical Association* 1993;269:2116–2121.

Fichhoff B. Why cancer communication can be hard. *Journal of National Cancer Institute Monographs* 1999;25:7–13.

Fineberg HV, Hiatt HH. Evaluation of medical practices. The case for technology assessment. *New England Journal of Medicine* 1979;301(20):1086–91.

Finucane ML, et al. The affect heuristic in judgments of risks and benefits. *Journal of Behavioral Decision Making* 2000;13:1–17.

Fong GT, Rempel LA, Hall PA. Challenges to improving health risk communication in the 21st century: a discussion. *Journal of National Cancer Institute Monographs* 1999;25:173–176.

Foote SB. Why Medicare cannot promulgate a national coverage rule: a case of regula mortis. *Journal of Health Politics, Policy and Law* 2002;27(5):707–729.

Foote SB. Focus on locus: evolution of Medicare's local coverage policy. *Health Affairs* 2003;22(4):137–146.

Fox DM, Leichter HM. Rationing care in Oregon: The new accountability. *Health Affairs* 1991;10(2):7–27.

Fox DM, Leichter HM. The ups and downs of Oregon's rationing plan. *Health Affairs* 1993;12(2):66–70.

Freemantle N, and Mason J. Publication bias in clinical trials and economic analyses. *Pharmacoeconomics* 1997;12(1):10–16.

Freudenheim M. Large H.M.O. to Make Treatment Guidelines Public. *New York Times* January 24, 2003, C3.

Friedberg M, Saffran B, Stinson TJ, Nelson W, Bennett CL. Evaluation of conflict of interest in economic analyses of new drugs used in oncology. *Journal of the American Medical Association* 1999;282:1453–1457.

Fryback DG, Dasbach EJ, Klein R, Klein BEK, Dorn N, Peterson K, Martin PA.

The Beaver Dam Health Outcomes Study: Initial catalog of health-state quality factors. *Medical Decision Making* 1993;13:89–102.

Gabriel SE, Kneeland TS, Melton LJ, Moncur MM, Ettinger B, Tosteson ANA. 1999. Health-related quality of life in economic evaluation of osteoporosis. *Medical Decision Making* 19:141–148.

Gafni A, Birch S. 1993. Economics, health and health economics: HYEs versus QALYs. *Journal of Health Economics* 11:325–39.

Gagnon JP. Sources of bias in the economic analyses of new drugs (letter to editor). *Journal of the American Medical Association* 2000;283:1423.

Galvin R, Milstein A. Large employers' new strategies in health care. *New England Journal of Medicine* 2002;19;347(12):939–942.

Gandek B, Ware JE, Aaronson NK, Apolone G, Bjorner JB, Brazier JE, Bullinger M, Kaasa S, Leplege A, Prieto L, Sullivan M. Cross-validation of item selection and scoring for the SF-12 Health Survey in nine countries: Results from the IQOLA Project. *Journal of Clinical Epidemiology* 1998;51(11):1171–1178.

Garber S, Ridgely MS, Taylor RS, Meili R. *Managed care and the evaluation and adoption of emerging medical technologies.* Rand: Santa Monica, 2000.

Garber AM. Realistic rigor in cost-effectiveness methods (Comment). *Medical Decision Making* 1999;19:378–79.

Garber AM. Evidence-based coverage policy. *Health Affairs* 2001;20(5):62–82.

Garber AM, Phelps CE. Economic foundations of cost-effectiveness analysis. *Journal of Health Economics* 1997;16(1):1–31.

Garrison LP, Wilensky GR. Cost containment and incentives for technology. *Health Affairs* 1983;(Summer)3:46–58.

Gaspoz JM, Coxson PG, Goldman PA, et al. Cost effectiveness of aspirin, clopidogrel, or both for secondary prevention of coronary heart disease. *New England Journal of Medicine* 2002;346(23):1800–1806.

George B, Harris A, Mitchell A. Cost-effectiveness analysis and the consistency of decision making: Evidence from pharmaceutical reimbursement in Australia (1991 to 1996). *Pharmacoeconomics* 2001;19(11):1103–1109.

Gerard K. Cost-utility in practice: A policy maker's guide to the state of the art. *Health Policy* 1992;21:249–279.

Gerard K, Smoker I, Seymour J. Raising the quality of cost-utility analyses: Lessons learnt and still to learn. *Health Policy* 1999;46:217–38.

Ginsberg ME, Kravitz RL, Sandberg WA. A survey of physician attitudes and practices concerning cost-effectiveness in patient care. *West Journal of Medicine* 2000;173:390–393.

Glick HA, Polsky D, Willke RJ, and Schulman KA. 1999. A comparison of preference assessment instruments used in a clinical trial. *Medical Decision Making* 19:265–275.

Gold MR, Siegel JE, Russell LB, Weinstein MC. *Cost-effectiveness in health and medicine.* Oxford University Press: Oxford, 1996.

Gold MR, Franks P, McCoy KI, Fryback DG. Toward consistency in cost-utility analyses: Using national measures to create condition-specific values. *Medical Care* 1998;36(6):778–92.

Gold M. Markets and public programs: insights from Oregon and Tennessee. *Journal of Health Politics, Policy, and Law* 1997;22(2):633–66.

Gold M. The changing U.S. health care system. *Milbank Quarterly* 1999;77:3–32.

Goldman L, Weinstein MC, Goldman PA, et al. Cost-effectiveness of HMG-CoA reductase inhibition for primary and secondary prevention of coronary heart disease. *Journal of the American Medical Association* 1991;265:1145–1151.

Goldsmith J. The road to meaningful reform: A conversation with Oregon's John Kitzhaber. *Health Affairs* 2003;22(1):114–124.

Gorham P. Cost-effectiveness guidelines: The experience of Australian manufacturers, *Pharmacoeconomics* 1995;8:369–373.

Grabowski H, Mullins CD. Pharmacy benefit management, cost-effectiveness analysis, and drug formulary decisions. *Society of Science and Medicine* 1997;45(4):535–544.

Grabowski H. The role of cost-effectiveness analysis in managed care decisions. *Pharmacoeconomics* 1998;14(Suppl 1):15–24.

Graham JD. Legislative approaches to achieving more protection at less cost. The University of Chicago Legal Forum: Chicago, 1997.

Graham JD, Corso PS, Morris JM, Segui-Gomez M, Weinstein MC. Evaluating the cost-effectiveness of clinical and public health measures. *Annual Review of Public Health* 1998;19:125–152.

Graham JD, Wiener JB. *Risk vs. Risk: Tradeoffs in protecting health and the environment.* Harvard University Press: Cambridge, MA, 1999.

Greenberg D, Pliskin JS. Preference-based outcome measures in cost-utility analyses. *International Journal of Technology Assessment in Health Care* 2002;18(3):461–466.

Greenberg D, Rosen AB, Olchanski NV, Stone PW, Nadai J, Neumann PJ. *Delays in publication of cost-utility analyses conducted alongside clinical trials.* BMJ 2004;328:1536–1537.

Grizzle AJ, Motheral BR, Olson BM. A qualitative assessment of managed care decision-makers' views and use of pharmacoeconomic information (abstract). *Value in Health* 2000;3(2):162.

Gross C, Anderson G, Powe N. The relation between funding by the National Institutes of Health and the burden of disease. *New England Journal of Medicine* 1999;340:1881–1887.

Gurm HS, Litaker DG. Framing procedural risks to patients: Is 99% safe the same as a risk of 1 in 100? *Academy of Medicine* 2000;75:840–842.

Haber SG, Khatutsky G, and Mitchell JB. Covering uninsured adults through Medicaid: Lessons from the Oregon health plan. *Health Care Financing Review* 2000;22(2):119–35.

Haddix AC, Teutsch SM, Shaffer PA, Dunet DO, eds. *Prevention effectiveness.* Oxford University Press: Oxford, England, 1996.

Hadorn DC. Setting health care priorities in Oregon: Cost-effectiveness meets the rule of rescue. *Journal of the American Medical Association* 1991;265:2218–2225.

Hadorn DC. The problem of discrimination in health care priority setting. *Journal of the American Medical Association* 1992;268:1454–1459.

Hahn RW. *Reviving regulatory reform: A global perspective.* American Enterprise Institute–Brookings Joints Center for Regulatory Studies: Washington D.C., 2000.

Hahn WR, Burnett JK, Chan YI, Mader EA, Moyle PR. Assessing regulatory impact analyses: The failure of agencies to comply with Executive Order 12,866. *Harvard Journal of Law and Public Policy* 2000;23(3):859–872.

Hahn RW, Dudley PM. Bush regulatory czar deserves high marks. *Policy Matters.* American Enterprise Institute–Brookings Joints Center for Regulatory Studies: Washington D.C., January 2002.

Hahn RW, Dudley PM, Irwin EL. Have government cost-benefit analyses improved over time? Working paper. American Enterprise Institute–Brookings Joints Center for Regulatory Studies: Washington D.C., September 20, 2002.

Hall MA. Legal challenges to managed care: Another view (letter to editor). *Health Affairs* 1999;18(6):246–247.

Ham C. Retracing the Oregon trail: The experience of rationing and the Oregon health plan. *British Medical Journal* 1998;316:1965–1969.

Hanley N, Spash CL. *Cost-benefit analysis and the environment.* Edward Elgar Publishing Company: Brookfield, VT, 1993.

Hardin G. The tragedy of the commons. *Science* 1968;1243–1248.

Harvard School of Public Health. The CEA Registry: Standardizing the Methods and Practices of Cost-effectiveness Analysis. Available at http://www.hsph.harvard.edu/cearegistry, 2002.

Hastie R, Viscusi WK. What juries can't do well: The jury's performance as a risk manager. *Arizona Law Review* 1998;40:901–921.

Hatziandreu E, Graham J, Stoto M. AIDS and biomedical research funding: Comparative analysis. *Reviews of Infectious Diseases* 1988;10:159–167.

Healthy People 2010. Available at http://www.healthypeople.gov/LHI/lhiwhat.htm. Accessed May 7, 2003.

Heinzerling L and Ackerman F. Pricing the priceless: Cost-benefit analysis of environmental protection. Georgetown Environmental Law and Policy Institute, Georgetown University Law Center: Washington, D.C. 2002.

Herrier RN, Boyce RW. Communicating risks to patients. *American Pharmacology* 1995;NS35:12–14.

Hershey J, Asch AD, Jepson C, Baron J, Ubel PA. Incremental and average cost-effectiveness ratios: Will physicians make a distinction? *Risk Analysis* 2003 Feb;23(1):81–89.

Hiatt HH. Protecting the medical commons: Who is responsible? *New England Journal of Medicine* 1975;293:235–241.

Hill SR, Mitchell AD, Henry DA. Problems with the interpretation of pharmacoeconomic analyses: A review of submissions to the Australian Pharmaceutical Benefits Scheme. *Journal of the American Medical Association* 2000;283:2116–2121.

Hillman AL, Eisenberg JM, Pauly MV, Bloom BS, Glick H, Kinosian B, Schwartz JS. Avoiding bias in the conduct and reporting of cost-effectiveness research sponsored by pharmaceutical companies. *New England Journal of Medicine* 1991;324(19):1362–1365.

Himmelstein DU, Woolhandler S. The Oregon health plan [letter]. *The New England Journal of Medicine* 1998;338(6):395–396.

Hirth RA, Chernew ME, Miller E, Fendrick AM, Weissert WG. Willingness to pay for a quality-adjusted life year: In search of a standard. *Medical Decision Making* 2000;20:332–342.

Hjelmgren J, Berggren F, Andersson F. Health economic guidelines—Similarities, differences, and some implications. *Value in Health* 2001;4(3):225–250.

Hoffman C, Stoykova BA, Nixon J, et al. Do health-care decision makers find economic evaluations useful? The findings of focus group research in U.K. health authorities. *Value in Health* 2002;5(2):71–78.

Hornberger JC, Redelmeier DA, Petersen J. 1992. Variability among methods to assess patients' well-being and consequent effect on a cost-effectiveness analysis. *Journal of Clinical Epidemiology* 45(5):505–512.

Howell J. Where is the NHS commissioning view in NICE decisions? (letter to editor) *British Medical Journal* 2001. March 13, 2001.

Hutubessy RCW, Balthussen RMPM, Evans DB, Barendregt JJ, Murray CJL. Stochastic league tables: Communicating cost-effectiveness results to decision makers. *Health Economics* 2001;10:473–477.

Hutubessy R, Baltussen R, Torres-Edejer TT, Evans DB. Generalised cost-effectiveness analysis: An aid to decision making in health. *Applied Health Economics and Health Policy* 2002;1(2):89–95.

Iglehart JK. The Centers for Medicare and Medicaid Services. *New England Journal of Medicine* 2001;345:1920–1924.

Iglehart JK. Changing health insurance trends. *New England Journal of Medicine* 2002;347(12):956–962.

Jackson BR, Busch MP, Stramer SL, AuBuchon JP. The cost-effectiveness of NAT for HIV, HCV, and HBV in whole-blood donations. *Transfusion* 2003 Jun;43(6): 721–729.

Jacobs L, Marmor T, Oberlander J. The Oregon health plan and the political paradox of rationing: What advocates and critics have claimed and what Oregon did. *Journal of Health Politics, Policy, and Law* 1999;24(1):161–180.

Jacobson PD, Rosenquist J. The introduction of low-osmolar contrast agents in radiology. *Journal of the American Medical Association* 1988;260:1586–1592.

Jacobson PD. Legal challenges to managed care cost containment programs: an initial assessment. *Health Affairs* 1999;18(4):69–85.

Jacobson PD, Kanna ML. Cost-effectiveness analysis in the courts: Recent trends and future prospects. *Journal of Health Policy, Politics, and Law* 2001;26(2):291–326.

Jamison DT et al., eds. *Disease control priorities in developing countries.* Oxford University Press: New York, 1993.

Janset SJT, Stiggelbout AM, Wakker PP et al. 1998. Patients' utilities for cancer treatments: A study of the chained procedure for the standard gamble and time tradeoff. *Medical Decision Making* 18:391–399.

Jefferson T, Demicheli V. Are guidelines for peer-reviewing economic evaluations necessary? A survey of current editorial practices. *Health Economics* 1995;4:383–388.

Jefferson TO, Smith R, Yee Y, Drummond MJ, Pratt M, Gale R. Evaluating the *BMJ* guidelines for economic submissions. *Journal of the American Medical Association* 1998;280:275–277.

Jefferson T, Demicheli V. Quality of economic evaluations in health care. *British Medical Journal* 2002;324:313–313.

Jefferson T, Demicheli V, Vale L. Quality of systematic reviews of economic evaluations in health care. *Journal of the American Medical Association* 2002;287:2809–2812.

Johannesson M and Jonsson B. Willingness to pay for antihypertensive therapy: Results of a Swedish pilot study. *Journal of Health Economics* 1991;10:461–474.

Johannesson M, Pliskin J, Weinstein M. 1993. Are healthy-years equivalents an improvement over quality-adjusted life years? *Medical Decision Making* 13(4):281–286.

Johannesson M. *Theory and methods of economic evaluation of health care.* Kluwer: Amsterdam, 1996.

Jstreetdata Fast Alert Study. Attitudes towards adoption of the AMCP formulary guidelines. November 2, 2001. Jstreetdata: Washington, D.C.

Kaiser Commission on Medicaid and the Uninsured. Oregon's Medicaid PDL: Will an evidence-based formulary with voluntary compliance set a precedent for Medicaid? Henry J. Kaiser Family Foundation: Washington, D.C., January 2004.

Kamm FM. To whom? *Hastings Center Report* 1994;24(4):29–32.

Kaplan RM, Anderson JP, Wu AW, Matthews WC, Kozin F, Orenstein D. 1989. The Quality of Well-Being Scale: Applications in AIDS, cystic fibrosis, and arthritis. *Medical Care* 27(3 Suppl):S27–S43.

Kassirer J, Angell M. The *Journal*'s policy on cost-effectiveness analyses. *New England Journal of Medicine* 1994;331:669–670.

Kaufman W. Oregon struggles to save health plan. National Public Radio broadcast, July 8, 2003.

Keith A. The economics of Viagra. *Health Affairs* 2000;19(2):147–157.

Kessler D, Pines W. The federal regulation of prescription drug advertising and promotion. *Journal of the American Medical Association* 1990;264(18):2409–2415.

Kilborn PT. Oregon falters on a new path to health care. *New York Times,* January 3, 1999, p. A1.

Kim M, Blendon RJ, Benson JM. How interested are Americans in new medical technologies? A multicountry comparison. *Health Affairs* 2001;5:194–201.

King R. Bitter pill: How a drug company paid for university study, then undermined it. *Wall Street Journal* April 25, 1996, p. A1.

Klarman HE. Cost-effectiveness analysis applied to treatment of chronic renal disease. *Medical Care* 1968;6:48–64.

Kmietowicz Z. Reform of NICE needed to boost its credibility. *British Medical Journal* 2001;323:1324.

Koepp R, Miles SH. Meta-analysis of tacrine for Alzheimer disease: The influence of industry sponsors. *Journal of the American Medical Association* 24 (1999):2287.

Kolata G. Newest treatments create a quandary on Medicare costs. *New York Times,* August 17, 2003, p. A1.

Kowalczyk L. Drug costs still ensnare health plans. *Boston Globe,* August 29, 2002, p. A1.

Krimsky S. Rothenberg LS. Financial interest and its disclosure in scientific publications. *Journal of the American Medical Association* 280 (1998):225–226.

Kuntz KM, Tsevat J, Weinstein MC, Goldman L. Expert panel vs. decision-analysis recommendations for postdischarge coronary angiography after myocardial infarction. *Journal of the American Medical Association* 1999;282:2246–2251.

Lagnado L. What is a bet on life worth? *Wall Street Journal,* June 18, 2003a, p. B1.

Lagnado L. Last hope for lymphoma, $28,000 a dose. *Wall Street Journal,* June 18, 2003b, p. B1.

Langley PC. Is cost-effectiveness modeling useful? *American Journal of Managed Care.* 2000;6(2):250–251.

Langley PC, Sullivan SD. Pharmacoeconomic evaluations: Guidelines for drug purchasers. *Journal of Managed Care Pharmacy* 1996;6(2):671–677.

Laupacis A, Wong C, Churchill D, and the Canadian Erythropoietin study group. The use of generic and specific qualty-of-life measures in hemodialysis patients treated with erythropoietin. *Controlled Clinical Trials* 1991;12:168S–179S.

Laupacis A, Feeny D, Detsky AS, Tugwell PX: How attractive does a new technology have to be to warrant adoption and utilization? Tentative guidelines for using clinical and economic evaluations. *Canadian Medical Association Journal* 1992;14:473–481.

Laupacis A. Inclusion of drugs in provincial drug benefit programs: Who is making these decisions, and are they the right ones? *Canadian Medical Association Journal* 2002;166(1):44–47.

Leaf A. Cost effectiveness as a criterion for Medicare coverage. *New England Journal of Medicine* 1989;321(13):898–900.

Leichter HM. Oregon's bold experiment: Whatever happened to rationing? *Journal of Health Politics, Policy, and Law* 1999;24(1):147–160.

Lemmens T, Singer PA. Bioethics for clinicians: Conflict of interest in research, education, and patient care. *Canadian Medical Association Journal* 159 (1998):960–965.

Lenert LA, Cher DJ, Goldstein MK, Bergen MR, and Garber A. The effect of search procedures on utility elicitations. *Medical Decision Making* 1998;18:76–83.

Levinsky NG. Truth or consequences. [Sounding Board]. *New England Journal of Medicine* 1998;338:913–915.

Levit K, Smith C, Cowan C, Lazenby H, Sensenig A, Catlin A. Trends in U.S. health care spending, 2001. *Health Affairs* 2003;22(1):154–164.

Lipman T. NICE and evidence-based medicine are not really compatible. (Letter to editor). *British Medical Journal* 2001;322:489.

Litvak E, Long MC, Schwartz JS. Cost-effectiveness analysis under managed care: Not yet ready for prime time? *American Journal of Managed Care* 2000;6(2):254–256.

Llewellyn-Thmas H, Sutherland HJ, Tibshirani R, Ciampi A, Till JE, Boyd NF. Describing health states. Methodologic issues in obtaining values for health states. *Medical Care* 1984;22:543–552.

Luce BR, Lyles AC, and Rentz AM. The view from managed care pharmacy. *Health Affairs* 1996;4:168–176.

Lyles A. Decision-makers' use of pharmacoeconomics: What does the research tell us? *Expert Rev. Pharmacoeconomics Res.* 2001;1(2):133–144.

Martinez B. Firms paid to trim drug costs also toil for drug makers. *Wall Street Journal* August 14, 2002, p. A1.

Mason J, Drummond M, Torrance G. Some guidelines on the use of cost-effectiveness league tables. *British Medical Journal* 1993;306:570–72.

Mason JM. Cost-per-QALY league tables: Their role in pharmacoeconomic analysis. *Pharmacoeconomics.* 1994;5:472–481.

Mathematica Policy Research. The role of PBMs in managing drug costs: Implications for a Medicare drug benefit. Report for the Henry J. Kaiser Family Foundation, January 2000.

Mather DB, Sullivan SD, Augenstein D, et al. Incorporating clinical outcomes into drug formulary decisions: A practical approach. *American Journal of Managed Care* 5:277–285.

Mauskopf J, Rutten F, Schonfeld W. Cost-effectiveness league tables: Valuable guidance for decision makers? *Pharmacoeconomics* 2003;21(14):991–1000.

Mayor S. NICE estimates that its recommendations have cost the NHS L575m. *British Medical Journal* 2002;325:924.

McGregor M. Cost-utility analysis: An instrument that should only be used with great caution. *Canadian Medical Association Journal* 2003;168(4):433–434.

McNeil BJ, Pauker SG, Sox HC, et al. On the elicitation of preferences for alternative therapies. *New England Journal of Medicine* 1982;306:1259–1262.

Mears R, Taylor R, Littlejohns P, Dillon A. Review of International Health Technology Assessment (IHTA). National Institute for Clinical Excellence, London. 2002.

Mechanic D. Muddling through elegantly: Finding the proper balance in rationing. *Health Affairs* 1997;16(5):83–92.

Medicare Prescription Drug, Improvement, and Modernization Act of 2003, Pub. L. no. 108–173, 117 Stat 2066 (2003).

Mehrez A, Gafni A. Quality adjusted life years, utility theory, and healthy-years equivalents. *Medical Decision Making* 1989;9(2):142–149.

Mehrez A and Gafni A. 1993. Healthy-years equivalents versus quality-adjusted life years: In pursuit of progress. *Medical Decision Making* 13:287–292.

Mello JJ, Brennan TA. The controversy over high-dose chemotherapy with autologous bone marrow transplant for breast cancer. *Health Affairs* 2001;20(5):101–117.

Meltzer D, Johannesson J. Inconsistencies in the "societal perspective" on costs of the Panel on Cost-Effectiveness in Health and Medicine. *Medical Decision Making* 1999;19:371–377.

Menon D, Schubert F, Torrance GW. Canada's new guidelines for the economic evaluation of pharmaceuticals. *Medical Care* 1996;34:DS77–DS86.

Merrill RA. Modernizing the FDA: An incremental revolution. *Health Affairs* 1999;18(2):96–111.

Messori A, Trippoli S, Daealessandro, Di Giorgio D, Tosolini F. Problems in pharmacoeconomic analyses (letter to editor). *Journal of the American Medical Association* 2000;284(15):1923.

Michaud C, Murray C, Bloom B. Burden of disease-implications for future research. *Journal of the American Medical Association* 2001;285:535–539.

Mishan EJ. Evaluation of life and limb. A theoretical approach. *Journal of Political Economy* 1971;79:687–706.

Mitchell A. Update and evaluation of Australian guidelines. *Medical Care* 1996;34: DS216–DS225.

Mitchell AS. Antipodean assessment: Activities, actions, and achievements. *International Journal of Technology Assessment in Health Care* 2002;18(2):203–212.

Mitchell JB, Bentley F. Impact of Oregon's priority list on Medicaid beneficiaries. *Medical Care Research and Review* 2000;57(2):216–234.

Mitchell JB, Haber SG, Khatutsky G, and Donoghue S. Impact of the Oregon health plan on access and satisfaction of adults with low income. Health Services Research 2002a;37(1):11–32.

Mitchell JB, Haber SG, Khatutsky G, Donoghue S. Children in the Oregon health plan: How have they fared? *Medical Care Research and Review* 2002b;59(2):166–183.

Mittmann N, Trakas K, Iskedjian M, Bradley CA, Einarson TR. A proposal for structured abstracts of health economic studies. *Annals of Pharmacotherapy* 1998;32:1244–1246.

Mohr P, Neumann PJ, Bausch S. Paying for new medical technology: Lesson for the Medicare program from other large health-care purchasers. Report for the Medicare Payment Advisory Commission. Project HOPE, Bethesda, MD. September 9, 2002.

Morris J, Hammitt JK. Using life expectancy to communicate benefits of health care programs in contingent valuation studies. *Medical Decision Making* 2001; 21(6):468–478.

Morrison GC. 1997. Healthy years equivalent and time tradeoff. What is the difference? *Journal of Health Economics* 16:563–578.

Morrow RH. Bryant JH. 1995. Health policy approaches to measuring and valuing human life: Conceptual and ethical issues. *American Journal of Public Health* 85(10):1356–1360.

Motheral BR, Grizzle AJ, Armstrong EP, Cox E, Fairman K. Role of pharmacoeconomics in drug benefit decision-making: Results of a survey. *Formulary* 2000;35(5):412–421.

Motheral B. Assessing the value of the Quality of Health Economic Studies (QHES) (editorial). *Journal of Managed Care Pharmacy* 2003;9(1):86–87.

Murray CJL. 1994. Quantifying the burden of disease: The technical basis for disability-adjusted life years. *Bulletin of the World Health Organization* 72(3):429–445.

Murray CJL and Lopez AD. *The global burden of disease*. World Health Organization: Geneva, Switzerland, 1996.

Murray CJL, Evans DB, Acharya A, Balthussen RMPM. Development of WHO guidelines on generalized cost-effectiveness analysis. *Health Economics* 2000;9: 235–251.

Nakao MA, Axelrod S. Numbers are better than words: Verbal specifications of frequency have no place in medicine. *American Journal of Medicine* 1983;74:1061–1065.

National Cancer Institute, 2001 Cancer Progress Report. Available at http://progressreport.cancer.gov/doc.asp?pid=1&did=21&chid=13&coid=33&mid=vpco. Accessed on January 17, 2004.

National Committee for Quality Assurance. Desirable Attributes of HEDIS Measures. NCQA, Washington DC. January 1998.

National Cholesterol Education Program (NCEP). The Second Report of the Expert Panel on Detection, Evaluation, and Treatment. *Circulation* 1994;89:1329–1445.

National Institute for Clinical Excellence. See www.nice.org.uk. Accessed August 3, 2003a.

National Institute for Clinical Excellence. See http://www.nice.org.uk/cat.asp?c=27588. Accessed September 18, 2003b.

National Highway Traffic Safety Administration. NHTSA Administrator Ricardo Martinez, M.D., will leave NHTSA and return to the private sector. Press release, September 30, 1999.

Navarro RP, Blackburn SS. Pharmacy benefit management companies. In Navarro RP, ed., *Managed care pharmacy practice*. Aspen Publications: Gaithersburg, MD, 1999, pp. 221–242.

Naylor CD, Chen E, Strauss B. Measured enthusiasm: Does the method of reporting trial results alter perceptions of therapeutic effectiveness? *Annals of Internal Medicine* 1992;117:916–921.

Nease RF Jr, Kneeland T, O'Conner GT, et al. Variation in patient utilities for outcomes of the management of chronic stable angina: Implications for clinical practice guidelines. *Journal of the American Medical Association* 1995:273:1185–1190.

Neuhauser D, Lewicki AM. What do we gain from the sixth stool guaiac? *New England Journal of Medicine* 1975;293:226–228.

Neumann PJ, Johannesson M. The willingness to pay for in vitro fertilization: A pilot study using contingent valuation. *Medical Care* 1994;32(7):686–699.

Neumann PJ, Zinner DE, and Paltiel AD. The FDA's regulation of cost-effectiveness claims. *Health Affairs* 1996;15(3):54–71.

Neumann PJ, Zinner DE, Wright JC. Are methods for estimating QALYs in cost-effectiveness analyses improving? *Medical Decision Making* 1997a;17:402–408.

Neumann PJ. Paying the piper for pharmacoeconomic studies. *Medical Decision Making* 1998;18(Suppl):S23–26.

Neumann PJ, Hermann RC, Kuntz KM. Cost effectiveness of donepezil in the treatment of mild or moderate Alzheimer's disease. *Neurology* 1999;52:1138–1145.

Neumann PJ, Stone PW, Chapman RH, Sandberg EA, Bell CM. The quality of reporting in published cost-utility analyses, 1976–1997. *Annals of Internal Medicine* 2000a;132:964–972.

Neumann PJ, Sandberg E, Bell C, et al. Are pharmaceuticals cost-effective? *Health Affairs* 2000b;19(2):92–109.

Neumann PJ, Claxton K, Weinstein MC. The FDA's regulation of health economic information. *Health Affairs* 2000c;19(5):129–37.

Neumann PJ, Goldie SJ, and Weinstein MC. Preference-based measures in economic evaluation of health care. *Annual Review of Public Health* 2000d;21:587–611.

Neumann PJ, Zivin KD, Ramakrishnan V, Stewart KA. Bell CM. Economic messages in prescription drug advertisements in leading medical journals. *Medical Care* 2002;40(9):840–845.

Neumann PJ, Levine BS. Do HEDIS measures reflect cost-effective practices? *American Journal of Preventive Medicine* 2002;23(4):276–289.

Neumann PJ. Evidence-based and value-based formulary guidelines. *Health Affairs* 2004a;23(1):124–134.

Neumann PJ. Why Don't Americans Use Cost-Effectiveness Analysis? *American Journal of Managed Care* 2004b;10(5):308–312.

Neumann PJ, Divi N, Beinfeld MT, Levine, Keenan P, Halpern EF, Gazelle GS. Quality of evidence and review times for Medicare national coverage decisions. Harvard School of Public Health. 2004.

Neumann PJ, Greenberg D, Olchanski NV, Stone PW, Rosen AB. Growth and quality of the cost-utility literature, 1976–2001. *Value in Health.* In press.

Nord E. 1992. An alternative to QALYs: The saved young life equivalent (SAVE). *British Medical Journal;* 305(6858):875–877.

——. Toward quality assurance in QALY calculations. *International Journal of Technology Assessment in Health Care* 1993a;9:37–45.

——. Unjustified use of the Quality of Well Being Scale in Oregon. *Health Policy* 1993b;24:45–53.

——. Health status index models for use in resource allocation decisions. *International Journal of Technology Assessment in Health Care* 1996;12:31–44.

——. *Cost-value analysis in health care.* Cambridge University Press: Cambridge UK, 1999.

O'Brien BJ, Drummond MF, Labelle RJ, Willan AR. In search of power and significance: Issues in the design and analysis of stochastic cost-effectiveness studies in health care. *Medical Care* 1994;32(2):150–163.

O'Brien BJ. Economic evaluation of pharmaceuticals: Frankenstein's monster or vampire of trials? *Medical Care* 1996;34(suppl):DS99–DS108.

O'Brien B, Gafni A. When do the "dollars" make sense? Toward a conceptual framework for contingent valuation studies in health care. *Medical Decision Making* 199616(3):288–299.

O'Brien BJ, Heyland D, Richardson WS, Levine M, Drummond MF, for the Evidence-Based Medicine Working Group. Users' guides to the medical literature: XIII. How to use an article on economic analysis: B. What are the results and will they help me in caring for my patients? *Journal of the American Medical Association* 1997;277:1802–1806.

O'Brien BJ, Goeree R, Hux M, et al. Economic evaluation of donepezil for the treatment of Alzheimer's disease in Canada. *Journal of the American Geriatric Society* 1999;47:520–578.

Ofman JJ, Sullivan SD, Neumann PJ, Chiou CF, Henning JM, Wade SW, Hay JW. Examining the value and quality of health economic analyses: Implications of utilizing the QHES. *Journal of Managed Care Pharmacy* 2003(9)1:53–61.

O'Grady MJ. The impact of regulatory and technological changes on the cost of inpatient blood and blood products: Implications for Medicare: Final report, submitted to Medicare Payment Advisory Commission. Project HOPE Center for Health Affairs: Bethesda, MD, November 6, 2001.

O'Leary JF, Faircloth DL, Jankowski MK, and Weeks JC. Comparison of time trade-off utilities and rating scale values of cancer patients and their relatives: Evidence for a possible plateau relationship. *Medical Decision Making* 1995;15: 132–137.

Olsen BM, Armstrong EP, Grizzle AJ, Nichter MA. Industry's Perception of Presenting Models to Managed Care Organizations. *Journal of Managed Care Pharmacy* 2003(9)2:159–167.

O'Riordan M. Reaction to Medicare ICD decision: Experts dismayed full MADIT II criteria not included in coverage. *Heartwire News* June 13, 2003.

Otrompke J. A new format for making more cost-effective drug coverage decisions takes off. *Business and Health* January 31, 2002.

Paltiel AD. Five minutes with the governor. *Medical Decision Making* 2000;20:239–242.

Patrick DL, Sittampalam Y, Somerville S, Carter W, Bergner M. A cross-cultural comparison of health status values. *American Journal of Public Health* 1985;75: 1402–1407.

Pauly MV. Valuing health care benefits in money terms. In Sloan F, ed. *Valuing Health Care* Cambridge University Press: Cambridge, U.K., 1995.

Pear R. Medicare to Weigh Cost as a Factor in Reimbursement. *The New York Times*, April 21, 1991, p. A1.

Pear R. Congress weighs drug comparisons: Pharmaceutical lobby opposes studies to rate prescriptions. *The New York Times*. August 24, 2003, p. A15.

Penna PM. AMCP Format for Formulary Submissions: Who is using them, who will be evaluating them, and what regulatory concerns do they raise? Presentation at the 7th Annual International Meeting of the International Society for Pharmacoeconomics and Outcomes Research, Arlington, VA, May 20, 2002.

Perneger TV, Martin DP, Bovier PA. Physicians' attitudes towards health care rationing. *Medical Decision Making* 2002;22:65–70.

Petrou S, Henderson J, Roberts T, Martin MA. Recent economic evaluations of antenatal screening: As systematic review and critique. *Journal of Medical Screening* 2000;7:59–73.

Pettiti D. *Meta-Analysis, decision analysis, and cost-effectiveness analysis: Methods for quantitative synthesis in medicine.* 2nd Edition. Oxford University Press: New York, 2000.

Phelps C, Parente S. Priority setting in medical technology and medical practice assessment. *Medical Care* 1990;28:703–723.

Phelps CE and Mushlin AI. On the (near) equivalence of cost-effectiveness and cost-benefit analysis. *International Journal of Technology Assessment in Health Care* 1991;7:12–21.

Phillips KA, Chen JL. Impact of the U.S. Panel on cost-effectiveness in health and medicine. *American Journal of Preventive Medicine* 2002;22(2):98–105.

Pignone M, Saha S, Hoerger T, Mandelblatt J. Cost-effectiveness analysis of colorectal cancer screening: A systematic review for the U.S. Prevention Services Task Force. *Annals of Internal Medicine* 2002;137:96–104.

The Pink Sheet. "Medicare Rx law would fundamentally change, not end, drug pricing debate. Chevy Chase, MD, June 16, 2003, p. 3.

Pinkerton SD, Johnson-Massotti AP, Holtgrave DR, Farnham PG. Using cost-effectiveness league tables to compare interventions to prevent sexual transmission of HIV. *AIDS* 2001;15:917–928.

Pinto JL, Lopez-Casasnovas G, and Ortun V, eds. *Economic evaluation: From theory to practice.* Springer-Verlag Iberica: Barcelona, Spain, 2001.

Pliskin JS, Shepard DS and Weinstein MC. 1980. Utility Functions for Life Years and Health Status. *Operations Research* 28(a):206–224.

Polsky D, Glick HA, Willke R, Schulman K. Confidence intervals for cost-effectiveness ratios: a comparison of four methods. *Health Economics* 1997;6(3): 243–252.

Powell M. Latest decision on zanamivir will not end postcode prescribing. *British Medical Journal* 2001;322:489.

Power EJ, Eisenberg JM. Are we ready to use cost-effectiveness analysis in health decision making? *Medical Care* 1998;36:MS10–17.

Prosser LA, Koplan JP, Neumann PJ, Weinstein MC. Barriers to using cost-effectiveness analysis in managed care decision making. *American Journal of Managed Care* 2000;6:173–179.

Pritchard C. Trends in economic evaluation. OHE Brief. Office of Health Economics, London. Paper No. 36, 1999.

Raferty J. NICE: faster access to modern treatment? Analysis of guidance on health technologies. *British Medical Journal* 2001;323:1300–1303.

Raiffa H. *Decision analysis.* Addison-Wesley: Reading, MA, 1968.

Ramsey SD, Etzioni R, Troxel A, and Urban N. Optimizing sampling strategies for estimating quality-adjusted life-years. *Medical Decision Making* 1997;17:431–38.

Ramsey SD, McIntosh M, Sullivan SD. Design issues for cost-effectiveness analyses alongside clinical trials. *Annual Review of Public Health* 2001;22:129–141.

Ramsey SD. Economic analyses and clinical practice guidelines: why not a match made in heaven? *Journal of General Internal Medicine* 2002;17(3): 235–237.

Rawlins MD. Reply from the chairman (Letter to editor). *British Medical Journal* 2001;322:489.

Read JL, Quinn RJ, Berwick DM, Fineberg HV, Weinstein MC. 1984. Preferences for health outcomes: comparison of assessment methods. *Medical Decision Making* 4:315–329.

Regalado A. To sell pricey drug, Eli Lilly fuels a debate over rationing. *Wall Street Journal* September 18, 2003, p. A1.

Regence Washington Health Pharmacy Service. Guidelines for Submission of Clinical and Economic Data Supporting Formulary Considerations, Version 1.2.

Regence Washington Health, University of Washington: Seattle, WA, September, 1997.

Regence Group. Formulary Submission Guidelines, Version 2.0. The Regence Group: Seattle, WA. 2002.

Reinhardt UE. Making economic evaluations respectable. *Social Science and Medicine* 1997;45:555–562.

Rennie D. Thyroid storm (editorial). *Journal of the American Medical Association* 1997;277:1238–1243.

Rennie D. Cost-effectiveness analysis: Making a pseudoscience legitimate. *Journal of Health Politics, Policy and Law* 2001;26(2):383–386.

Rennie D, Luft HS. Pharmacoeconomic analyses: Making them transparent, making them credible. *Journal of the American Medical Association* 2000;283:2158–2160.

Reuters Medical News. UK government acts to defuse MS drug row. October 31, 2001.

Revicki DA, Shakespeare A, and Kind P. Preferences for schizophrenia-related health states: A comparison of patients, caregivers, and psychiatrists. *International Clinical Psychopharmacology* 1996;11:101–108.

Reinhardt UE. Making economic evaluations respectable. *Social Science Medicine* 1997;45:555–562.

Remund D, Valentino MA. United States government experience with cost-effectiveness analysis in formulary review. Presentation at the Agency for Health Care Research and Quality, Rockville, MD, May 22, 2003.

Robinson JC. The end of managed care. *Journal of the American Medical Association.* 2001;285:2622–2628.

Robinson AM, AMCP's Format for Formulary Submissions: An evolving standard. Results of two recent surveys. Presentation at the 15th Annual Meeting of the Academy of Managed Care Pharmacy, Minneapolis, MN April 9–12, 2003.

Rochon PA, Gurwitz JH, Simms RW, et al. A study of manufacturer-supported trials of nonsteroidal anti-inflammatory drugs in the treatment of arthritis. *Archives of Internal Medicine* 154 (1994):157–163.

Rosen AB, Greenberg D, Stone PW, Olchanki WV, Nadai N, Neumann PJ. Quality of abstract reporting in cost-effectiveness analyses. Harvard School of Public Health: Cambridge, MA, 2003.

Rosenbaum S, Frankford DM, Moore B, Borzi P. Who should determine when health care is medically necessary? *New England Journal of Medicine* 1999;343: 229–232.

Russell LB. *Is prevention better than cure?* Brookings Institute: Washington, D.C., 1986.

Russell LB, Gold MR, Siegel JE, Daniels N. The role of cost-effectiveness analysis in health and medicine. *Journal of the American Medical Association* 1996;276: 1172–1177.

Russell LB. Improving the Panel's recommendations. (Comment). *Medical Decision Making* 1999;19:379–380.

Sackett D, Torrance G. The utility of different health states as perceived by the general public. *Journal of Chronic Diseases* 1978;31(11):697–704.

Sacramento HealthCare Decisions. Cost-effectiveness as a criterion for medical and coverage decisions: Understanding and responding to community perspectives. Rancho Cordova, CA, October 2001.

Saha S, Hoerger TJ, Pignone MP, et al. The art and science of incorporating cost effectiveness into evidence-based recommendations for clinical preventive services. *American Journal of Preventive Medicine* 2001;20(3S):36–43.

Samsa GP, Cohen SJ, Goldstein LB, et al. Knowledge of risk among patients at increased risk for stroke. *Stroke* 1997;28:916–921.

Sandberg EA, Neumann PJ, Thompson KM, Goldman PA, Weinstein MC. *Validating models for health policy decisions.* Harvard School of Public Health: Cambridge, MA, 2003.

Schauffler HH. Disease prevention policy under Medicare: A historical and political analysis. *American Journal of Preventive Medicine* 1993;9:71–7.

Schoonmaker MM, Bernhardt BA, Holtman NA. Factors influencing health insurers' decisions to cover new genetic technologies. *International Journal of Technology Assessment in Health Care* 2000;16:178–79.

Schulenburg J-M Graf v d, ed. *The influence of economic evaluation studies on health care decision making: A European survey.* IOS Press: Amsterdam, 2000.

Schulman K, Sulmasy DP, Roney D. Ethics, economics, and the publication policies of major medical journals. *Journal of the American Medical Association* 1994;272:154–156.

Sculpher M, Drummond M, O'Brien B. Effectiveness, efficiency, and NICE (editorial) *British Medical Journal* 2001;322:943–944.

Schelling TC. The life you save may be your own. In Bhase SB, ed. *Problems in Public Expenditure Analysis.* Brookings Institute: Washington, D.C., 1968:127–176.

Schwartz LM, Woloshin S, Black WC, Welch HG. The role of numeracy in understanding the benefit of screening mammography. *Annals of Internal Medicine* 1997;127:966–972.

Schwarz RP. Maintaining integrity and credibility in industry-sponsored research. *Controlled Clinical Trials* 12(1991):753–760.

Sheingold SH. Technology assessment, coverage decisions, and conflict: The role of guidelines. *American Journal of Managed Care* 1998;4:SP117–SP125.

Shekar SS. Health care coverage for Medicare: Cost-effectiveness of new technology. *Journal of Laparoendoscopic Surgery* 1993;3:383–387.

Siegel JE, Weinstein MC, Russell LB, Gold MR, for the Panel on Cost-Effectiveness in Health and Medicine. Recommendations for reporting cost-effectiveness analyses. *Journal of the American Medical Association* 1996;276:1339–1341.

Siegel J, Byron S, Lawrence W. Federal Sponsorship of Health Economics Research: 1997–2001. Agency for Health Care Research and Quality: Rockville, MD, 2003.

Singer PA. Resource allocation: Beyond evidence-based medicine and cost-effectiveness analysis. *ACP Journal Club* 1997;127:A16–18.

Singer S, Bergthold L, Vorhaus C, Olson S, Mutchnick I, Goh YY, Zimmerman S, Enthovan A. Decreasing variation in medical necessity decision making: Final report to the California HealthCare Foundation. Center for Health Policy: Stanford University, August 1999.

Singer SJ, Bergthold LA. Prospects for improved decision making about medical necessity. *Health Affairs* 2001;1:200–206.

Sloan FA, Whetten-Goldstein K, Wilson A. Hospital pharmacy decisions, cost-containment, and the use of cost-effectiveness analysis. *Social Science and Medicine* 1997;45(4):525–533.

Slovic P. Perception of risk. *Science* 1987;236:280–285.

Slovic P. Trust, emotion, sex, politics, and science. Surveying the risk-assessment battlefield. *Risk Analysis* 1999;19:689–701.

Smith R. The failings of NICE (editorial). *British Medical Journal* 2000;321:1363–1364.

Smith KJ, Roberts MS. Cost-effectiveness of sildenafil. *Annals of Internal Medicine* 2000;132:933–937.

Stalhammer NO and Johanesson M. Valuation of health changes with the contingent valuation method: A test of scope and question order effects. *Health Economics* 1996;5:531–541.

Starr P. *The social transformation of American medicine.* Basic Books, Inc.: New York, 1982.

Steiner C et al. The review process used by health care plans to evaluate new medical technology for coverage. *Journal of General Internal Medicine* 1996;11:294–302.

Stelfox HT, Chua G, O'Rourke KO, Detsky AS. Conflict of interest in the debate over calcium-channel antagonists. *New England Journal of Medicine* 338 (1998):101–106.

Stephenson J. Medical technology watchdog plays unique role in quality assessment. *Journal of the American Medical Association* 1995;274:999–1001.

Stergachis A. Format for formulary submissions: Challenges, opportunities, and expectations for industry. Presentation at the AMCP Educational Conference, Dallas, TX, Oct. 19, 2001.

Stewart KA, Neumann PJ. FDA actions against misleading or unsubstantiated economic and quality-of-life claims: An analysis of warning letters and notices of violation. *Value in Health* 2002;5(5):389–396.

Stinnett AA, Mullahy J. Net health benefits: A new framework for the analysis of uncertainty in cost-effectiveness analysis. *Medical Decision Making* 1998;18(Suppl):S68–S80.

Stone PW, Liljas B, Chapman RC, Sandberg EA, Bell C., and Neumann PJ. Variations in methods to estimate costs in cost-effectiveness analyses. *International Journal of Technology Assessment in Health Care* 2000;16(1):111–124.

Stoykova BA, Hoffman C, Drummond M, Glanville JM, Nixon J. Do decision makers find economic evaluations useful? Part II: Issues emerging from recent Western European studies. In Schulenburg J-M Graf v d, ed. *The influence of economic evaluation studies on health care decision making: A European survey.* IOS Press: Amsterdam, 2000.

Strongin R. Medicare coverage: Lessons from the past, questions for the future. National Health Policy Forum, Washington, DC, August 2001.

Strunk BC, Reschovsky JD. Kinder and gentler: Physicians and managed care,

1997–2001. Center for Studying Health System Change, Washington, DC, Vol. 5, November 2002.

Studdert DM, Gresenz CR. Enrollee appeals of pre-service coverage denials at 2 health maintenance organizations. *Journal of the American Medical Association* 2003;289:864–870.

Sullivan SD, Lyles A, Luce B, Gricar. AMCP guidance for submission of clinical and economic evaluation data to support formulary listing in U.S. health plans and pharmacy benefits management organizations. *Journal of Managed Care Pharmacy* 2001;7(4):272–282.

Task Force on Principles for Economic Analysis of Health Care Technology. Economic analysis of health care technology: A report on principles. *Annals of Internal Medicine* 1995;123:61–70.

Taylor D. Funding medicines for people with multiple sclerosis. *British Medical Journal* 2001;323:1379–1380.

Tengs TO, Adams ME, and Pliskin JS et al. Five-hundred life-saving interventions and their cost-effectiveness. *Risk Analysis* 1995;15:369–390.

Tengs TO, Meyer G, Siegel JE et al. "Oregon's Medicaid rankings and cost-effectiveness: Is there any relationship?" *Medical Decision Making* 1996;16:99–107.

Tengs TO, Graham JD. The opportunity costs of haphazard social investments in life-saving. In Hahn RW, ed. *Risks, costs, and lives saved.* Oxford University Press: Oxford, UK, 1996, pp. 167–182.

Thompson DF. Understanding financial conflicts of interest. *New England Journal of Medicine* 329 (1993):573–576.

Thompson KM, Segui-Gomez M, Graham JD. Validating benefit and cost estimates: The case of airbag regulation. *Risk Analysis* 2002;22(4):803–811.

Titlow K, Randel L, Clancy CM, Emanuel EJ. Drug coverage decisions: The role of dollars and values. *Health Affairs* 2000;19(2):240–247.

Toner R, Stolberg SG. Decades after health care crisis, soaring costs bring new strains. *New York Times*, August 11, 2002, p. A1.

Torrance GW, Thomas W, Sackett D. 1972. A utility maximization model for evaluation of health care programs. *Health Services Research* 7(2):118–133.

Torrance GW. 1976. Social preferences for health states: An empirical evaluation of three measurement techniques. *Socio-Economic Planning Sciences* 10;128–136.

Torrance GW, Boyle MH, and Horwood SP. 1982. Application of multi-attribute utility theory to measure social preferences for health states. *Operations Research* 30:1043–1069.

Torrance GW. 1986. Measurement of health state utilities for economic appraisal. *Journal of Health Economics* 5:1–30.

Torrance GW, Feeny DH, Furlong WJ, Barr RD, Zhang Y, Wang Q. 1996. Multi-attribute preference functions for a comprehensive health status classification systems: Health Utilities Index Mark 2. *Medical Care* 24(7):702–722.

Towse A., Pritchard C. Does NICE have a threshold? An external view? In Towse A, Pritchard C, Devlin N, eds. Cost-effectiveness Thresholds Economic and Ethical issues. OHE: London, 2002.

Tsevat J, Cook EF, Green ML, et al. Health values of the seriously ill. *Annals of Internal Medicine* 1995;122:514–520.

Tsevat J, Dawson MD, Wu AW et al. Health values of hospitalized patients 80 years old or older. *Journal of the American Medical Association* 1998;279;371–375.

Tsevat J, Solzan JG, Kuntz KM, et al. Health values of patients infected with human immunodeficiency virus: Relationship to mental health and physical functioning. *Medical Care* 1996;34:44–57.

Tunis SR, Kang JL. Improvements in Medicare coverage of new technology. *Health Affairs* 2001;20(5):83–85.

Tunis SR, Stryer DB, Clancy CM. Practical clinical trials: Increasing the value of clinical research for decision making in clinical and health policy. *Journal of the American Medical Association.* 2003;290;1624–1632.

Tversky A, Kahneman D. The framing of decisions and the psychology of choice. *Science* 1981;211:453–58.

Ubel PA, Loewenstein G. The efficacy and equity of retransplantation: An experimental survey of public attitudes. *Health Policy* 1995;34:145–51.

Ubel PA, Loewenstein G, Scanlon D. Kamlet M. Individual utilities are inconsistent with rationing choices: A partial explanation of why Oregon's cost-effectiveness list failed. *Medical Decision Making* 1996;16(2):108–116.

Ubel PA, Loewenstein G, Scanlon D, Kamlet M. Value measurement in cost-utility analysis: Explaining the discrepancy between analog scale and person trade-off elicitations. *Health Policy* 1998a:43:33–44.

Ubel PA, Spranca M, DeKay M, et al. Public preferences for prevention versus cure: What if an ounce of prevention is worth only an ounce of cure? *Medical Decision Making* 1998b;18:141–148.

Ubel PA. *Pricing life.* The MIT Press: Cambridge, MA, 2000.

Ubel PA, Baron J, Nash B, Asch DA. Are preferences for equity over efficiency in health care allocation "all or nothing"? *Medical Care* 2000;38:366–373.

Ubel PA, Jepson C, Baron J, Hershey JC, Asch DA. The influence of cost-effectiveness information on physicians' cancer screening recommendations. *Social Science and Medicine* 2003a;56(8):1727–1736.

Ubel PA, Hirth RA, Chernew ME, Fendrick AM. What is the price of life and why doesn't it increase at the rate of inflation? *Archives of Internal Medicine* 2003b;163:1637–41.

Udvarhelyi IS, Colditz GA, Rai A, Epstein AM. Cost-effectiveness and cost-benefit analyses in the medical literature: Are they being used correctly? *Annals of Internal Medicine* 1992;116:238–244.

U.S. 11th Circuit Court of Appeals. PHARMAC vs. Meadows, September 6, 2002.

U.S. Code: FDAMA, P.L. 105–115.

U.S.C. §1369r-8(d)(4). Medicaid Drug Rebate law . . . 42 U.S.C. §1369r-8(d)(4).

U.S. Congress, House of Representatives, Committee on Ways and Means, Subcommittee on Health. "Issues Relating to Medicare's Coverage Policy." April 17, 1997.

U.S. Congress. Conference Committee report elaborating on language pertaining to health care economic information in the Food and Drug Administration Modernization Act of 1997b.

U.S. Congress, Senate Labor and Human Resources Committee, Subcommittee on Public Health and Safety. Statement of Nancy-Ann Min DeParle, Administrator, Health Care Financing Administration. March, 12, 1998.

U.S. Congress, House of Representatives. H.R. 2356, "To require the National Institutes of Health to conduct research, and the Agency for Health Research and Quality to conduct studies, on the comparative effectiveness and cost-effectiveness of prescription drugs that account for high levels of expenditures or use by individuals in federally funded health programs, and for other purposes." June 5, 2003.

U.S. Federal Register. Medicare Program. Procedures for Medical Services Coverage Decisions; Request for Comments. April 29, 1987; Vol. 52 (No. 82); 15560–15563.

U.S. Federal Register. Medicare Program: Criteria and Procedures for Making Medical Services Coverage Decisions That Relate to Health Care Technology." 1989;54(30):4302–4318. January 30, 1989.

U.S. Federal Register. Medicare Program: Criteria and Procedures for Extending Coverage to Certain Medical Devices and Related Services. 1995;60(181):48417–48425. September 19, 1995 (42 CFR Parts 405 and 411).

U.S. Federal Register. Executive Order 12291. 46 FR 13193; February 17, 1981.

U.S. Federal Register. Executive Order 12866 regulatory planning and review. September 30, 1993. Vol. 58, page 51735.

U.S. Federal Register. Medicare Program: Establishment of the Medicare Coverage Advisory Committee and Request for Nominations for Members. 1998; 63(239):68780. December 14, 1998.

U.S. Federal Register. Medicare Program: Procedures for Making National Coverage Decisions. 1999;64(80):22619–22625. April 27, 1999.

U.S. Federal Register Notice. Medicare Coverage Policy—Coverage Process. Criteria for Making Coverage Decisions. May 16, 2000. 2000:65(95):31124–31129.

U.S. Federal Register. Proposed Rule. Changes to the hospital inpatient prospective payment systems and fiscal year 2002 rates. May 4, 2001. Vol. 66, Number 87: 207–344.

U.S. Food and Drug Administration, Division of Drug Marketing, Advertising, and Communications, Principles for the Review of Pharmacoeconomic Promotion, Draft Guidelines. 1995.

U.S. Medicare Payment Advisory Commission. Accounting for new technology in hospital prospective payment systems. In Report to the Congress: Medicare Payment Policy. Washington, DC, March 2001, pp. 35–45.

U.S. Medicare Payment Advisory Commission. Paying for new technology in the outpatient prospective payment systems. Report to the Congress: Medicare Payment Policy. Washington, DC, March 2002, pp. 110–120.

U.S. Medicare Payment Advisory Commission. Report to the Congress on Assessing Medicare Benefits. Washington, DC, June 2002.

U.S. Office of Management and Budget. OSHA Prompt Letter from John D. Graham, Administrator of the Office of Information and Regulatory Affairs, OMB, to John Henshaw, Assistant Secretary of Labor, Occupational Safety and Health Administration, on the use of automated external defibrillators. September 18, 2001a.

U.S. Office of Management and Budget. HHS Prompt Letter. Letter from John D. Graham, Administrator of the Office of Information and Regulatory Affairs, OMB, to Tommy G. Thompson, Secretary of Health and Human Services, on the trans fatty acid rule. September 18, 2001b.

U.S. Office of Management and Budget. "OMB encourages lifesaving actions by regulators." Press release, September 18, 2001c.

U.S. Office of Management and Budget. Federal Budget Submission, 2002. Chapter 24: Ranking regulatory investments in public health.

U.S. Office of Management and Budget. Draft 2003 Report to Congress on the Costs and Benefits of Federal Regulations. February 3, 2003.

U.S. Office of Technology Assessment, The State of Cost-Effectiveness Analysis, in Identifying Health Technologies That Work, OTA-H-608. Washington, DC: U.S. Government Printing Office, September 1994, pp. 107–130.

U.S. Public Health Service, Office of Research, Statistics and Technology. Health: United States. Hyattsville, MD: U.S. Department of Health and Human Services, 1981.

Van Wijck EEE, Bosch JL, and Hunink MGM. Time-tradeoff values and standard gamble utilities assessed during telephone interviews versus face-to-face interviews. *Medical Decision Making* 1998;18:400–405.

Viscusi WK, The value of risks to life and health. *Journal of Economic Literature* 1993;31:1912–1946.

Vladeck BC. Commentary on Mitchell and Bentley, "Impact of Oregon's priority list on Medicaid beneficiaries." *Medical Care Research and Review* 2000;57(2):235–242.

Vogel VG. Tools for evaluating a patient's 50-year and lifetime probabilities. *Postgraduate Medicine* 1999;49–60.

Von-Neumann J and Morgenstern O. *Theory of games and economic behavior*. Princeton University Press: Princeton, NJ, 1994.

Walker R. "Spinning" is not NICE. (Letter to editor). *British Medical Journal* 2001;322:489.

Wallace JF, Weingarten SR, Chiou CF, et al. The limited incorporation of economic analyses in clinical practice guidelines. *Journal of General Internal Medicine* 2002;17:210–220.

Wakker P. 1996. A criticism of healthy years equivalents. *Medical Decision Making* 16:207–214.

Warner KE, Luce BR. *Cost-benefit and cost-effectiveness analysis in health care*. Health Administration Press: Ann Arbor, MI, 1982.

Weinstein MC, Stason WB. Foundations of cost-effectiveness analysis for health and medical practice. *New England Journal of Medicine* 1977;296:716–721.

Weinstein MC and Fineberg HV. *Clinical decision analysis*. W.B. Saunders Co: Philadelphia, 1980.

Weinstein M. Cost-effective priorities for cancer prevention. *Science* 1983;221:17–23.

Weinstein MC, Siegel JE, Gold MR, Kamlet MS, Russell LB, for the Panel on Cost-Effectiveness in Health and Medicine. Recommendations of the Panel on Cost-Effectiveness in Health and Medicine. *Journal of the American Medical Association.* 1996;276:1253–1258.

Weinstein MC. High-priced technology can be good value for money. *Annals of Internal Medicine* 1999;130(10):857–858.

Weinstein MC. Theoretically correct cost-effectiveness analysis (Comment). *Medical Decision Making* 1999;19:380–382.

Weinstein MC. Should physicians be gatekeepers of medical resources? *Journal of Medical Ethics* 2001a;27:268–274.

Weinstein MC, Toy E, Sandberg EA, Neumann PJ, Evans JS, Kuntz KM, Graham JD, Hammitt JK. Modeling for public policy decisions: Uses, roles, and validity. *Value in Health* 2001b;4:348–361.

Weinstein MC. We ration health care: Better to do it rationally. *Washington Post.* June 1, 2003, p. B3.

Weisbrod BA. *The economics of public health.* University of Pennsylvania Press: Philadelphia, 1961.

Willan AR, O'Brien BJ. Confidence intervals for cost-effectiveness ratios: An application of Feiller's theorem. *Health Economics* 1996;5(4):297–305.

Willems JS, Sanders CR, Riddiough MA, et al. Cost-effectiveness of vaccination against pneumococcal pneumonia. *New England Journal of Medicine* 1980;303:553–559.

Williams A. Intergenerational equity: An exploration of the "fair innings" argument. *Health Economics* 1997;6:117–132.

Williams A. The role of economics in evaluating health care. In Pinto JL, Lopez-Casasnovas G, and Ortun V, eds. *Economic evaluation: From theory to practice.* Springer-Verlag Iberica: Barcelona, Spain, 2001, pp. 3–16.

Winkelmeyer WC, Neumann PJ. *Cost-effective or not? Practices and recommendations for reporting cost-effectiveness thresholds in the literature.* Harvard School of Public Health: Cambridge, MA, 2002.

Winslow R, McGinley L, Adams C. States, insurers, find prescriptions for high drug costs. *Wall Street Journal.* September 11, 2002, p. A1.

Woloshin S, Schwartz LM, Byram S, et al. A new scale for assessing perceptions of chance: A validation study. *Medical Decision Making* 2000;20:298–307.

Wood AJ. When increased therapeutic benefit comes at increased cost. *New England Journal of Medicine* 2002; 346(23):1819–21.

World Bank. *World development report, 1993: Investing in health.* Oxford University Press: New York, 1993.

World Health Organization. *World Health Report 2002.* Available at http://www.who.int/whr/2002/en/. Accessed March 21, 2003.

World Health Organization. What is WHO-CHOICE? Available at www3.who.int/whosis/cea/guide/guide.cfm?path=whosis,cea,cea_guide&language=English. Accessed September 8, 2003.

Wright JC, Weinstein MC. Gains in life expectancy from medical interventions—standardizing data on outcomes. *New England Journal of Medicine* 1998;339:380–386.

Zellmer W. Comments of the American Society of Health-System Pharmacists. Presentation at the Food and Drug Administration Hearing, "Pharmaceutical Marketing and Information Exchange in Managed Care Environments." Silver Spring, MD, October 19, 1995.

Index

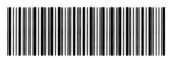